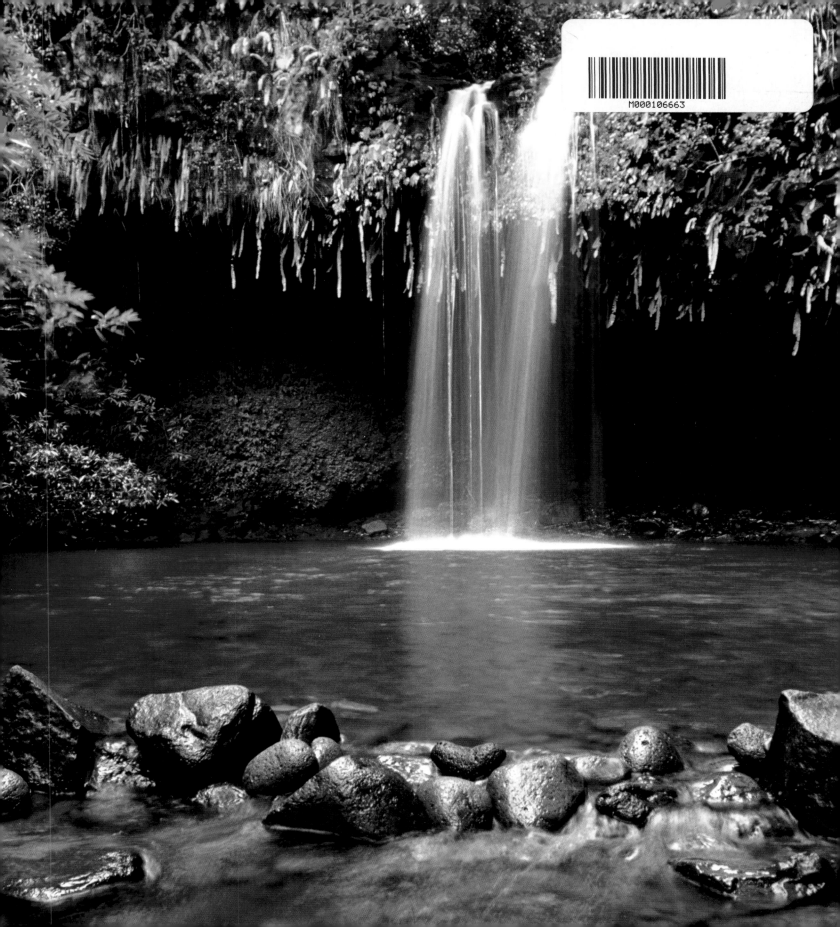

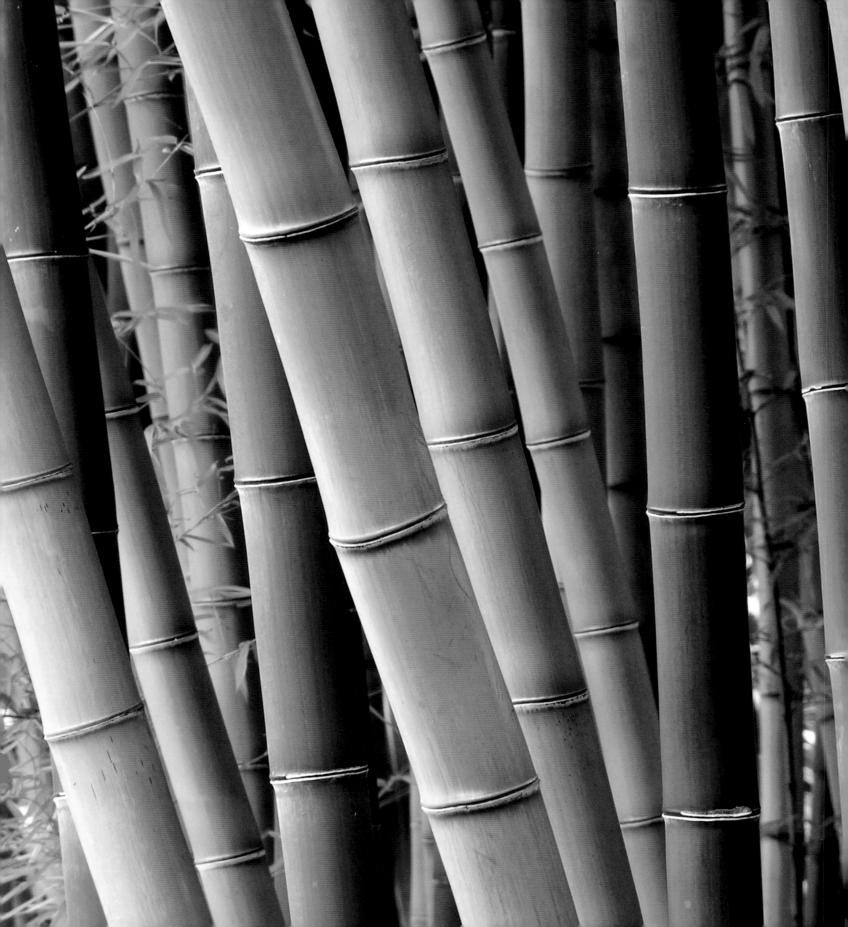

NURTURING BODY, MIND, AND SPIRIT

An Island Spa Experience

Cheryl Chee Tsutsumi

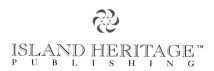

ISLAND HERITAGE™
PUBLISHING

An Island Spa Experience: Nurturing Body, Mind, and Spirit provides general information about health and healing. Although the book contains recipes and recommendations that have been shown to be helpful for preventing and alleviating certain health problems, it does not guarantee their effectiveness nor advocate their use.

Island Heritage Publishing, the author, photographers, and their heirs assume no liability for any conditions that may result from treatments described in this book. The information contained herein is not intended to replace advice you would receive from your doctor, pharmacist, and other health experts after a thorough review of your medical history.

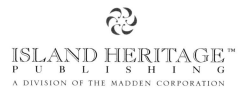

ISLAND HERITAGE™
P U B L I S H I N G
A DIVISION OF THE MADDEN CORPORATION

94-411 Kō'aki Street, Waipahu, Hawai'i 96797-2806
Orders: (800) 468-2800 • Information: (808) 564-8800
Fax: (808) 564-8877 • islandheritage.com

ISBN: 1-59700-156-2
First Edition, First Printing, 2008

table of contents

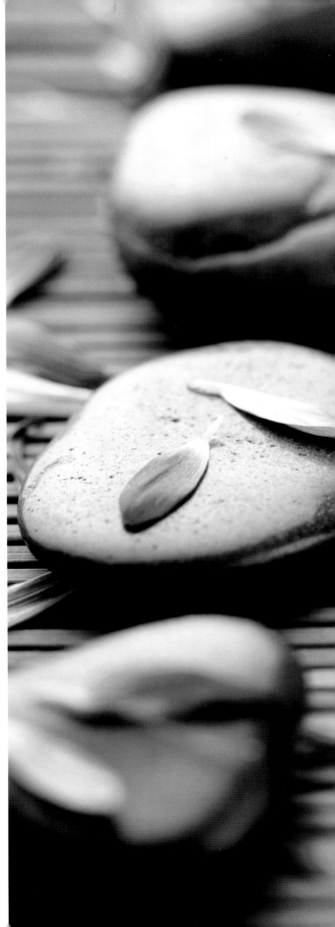

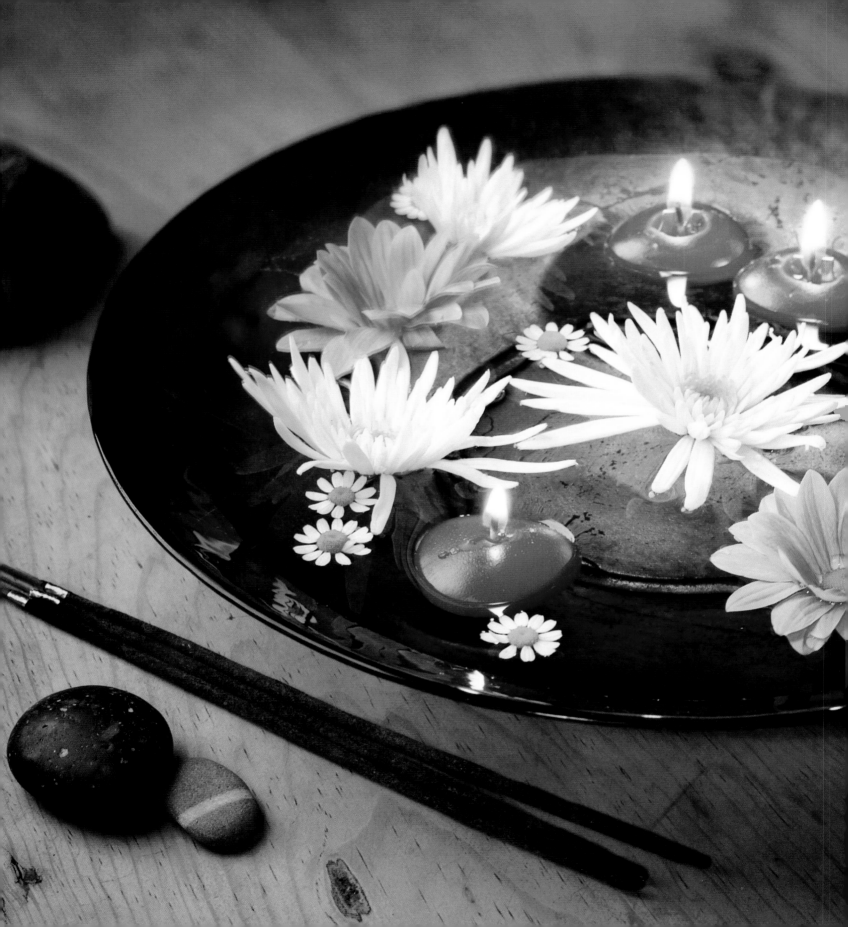

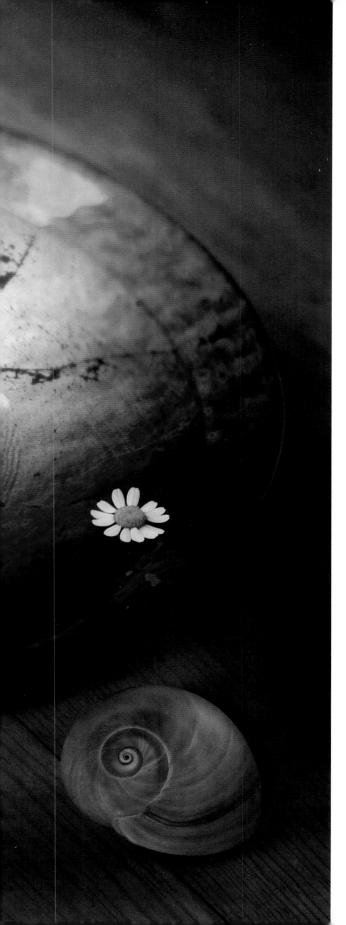

acknowledgments

I'd like to extend a special *mahalo* (thank-you) to the following people, who, through their wisdom, spirituality, and *aloha*, helped guide me on my own healing journey.

Patience Namaka Bacon

Mary Fragas

Kawaikapuokalani Hewett

Kai Keali'ikea'ehale O Kaholokai

Charles Ka'upu

Sylvester Kepilino

Nerita Machado

Clifford Nae'ole

Kapi'ioho'okalani Lyons Naone

Levon Ohai

Marie Place

Dane Ka'ohelani Silva

Dr. Laurie Steelsmith

Ramsay Taum

Dr. Jason Uchida

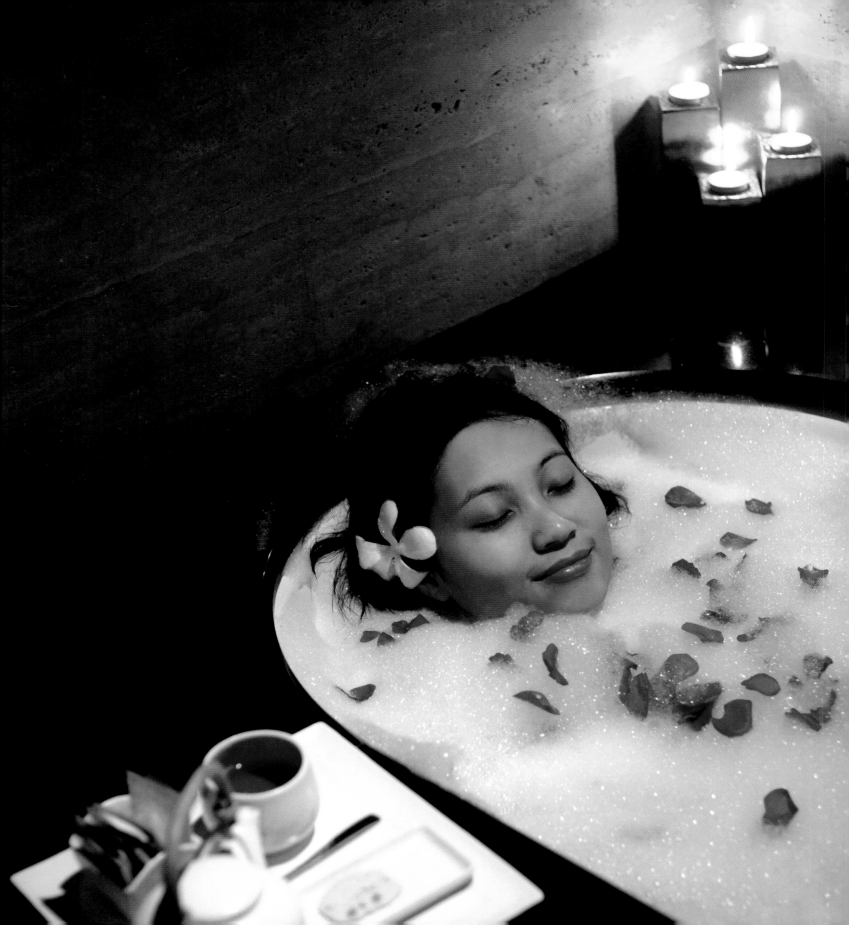

introduction

Aaahhh, the spa! The very word evokes images of hedonistic indulgences, of delightful diversions. In havens that are as still and lovely as a rain forest, your aches and pains melt away, peace fills your mind and body, and you're transported to the threshold of nirvana.

The modern spa, however, is no longer designed purely for pleasure. Treatments and classes on subjects such as conditioning, nutrition, meditation, and stress management help patrons achieve long-term health goals. Rather than just addressing physical symptoms, spas now champion a holistic philosophy.

An Island Spa Experience: Nurturing Body, Mind, and Spirit leads you on a path to total well-being that's influenced by ancient Hawaiian beliefs, practices, and traditions. It describes the beautification techniques and medicinal treatments of *ka po'e kahiko* (the people of old), and how they are being incorporated in spas today.

You'll learn about the history of the spa; discover extraordinary island treatments; meet renowned Native Hawaiian healing experts; and find out how touch, smell, sight, sound, taste, meditation, water, and exercise are being used to alleviate disease and discomfort.

The book concludes with a roundup of top spas statewide; health and beauty recipes you can easily make at home using ingredients in your kitchen; and a comprehensive list of resources, including holistic centers and wellness retreats, health- and fitness-related events, and manufacturers of quality spa products and accessories.

Hopefully, *An Island Spa Experience* will inspire, rejuvenate, and reward you with a renewed passion for life.

LEFT: A long soak in a bubble
bath is a great way to unwind.

old days, old ways

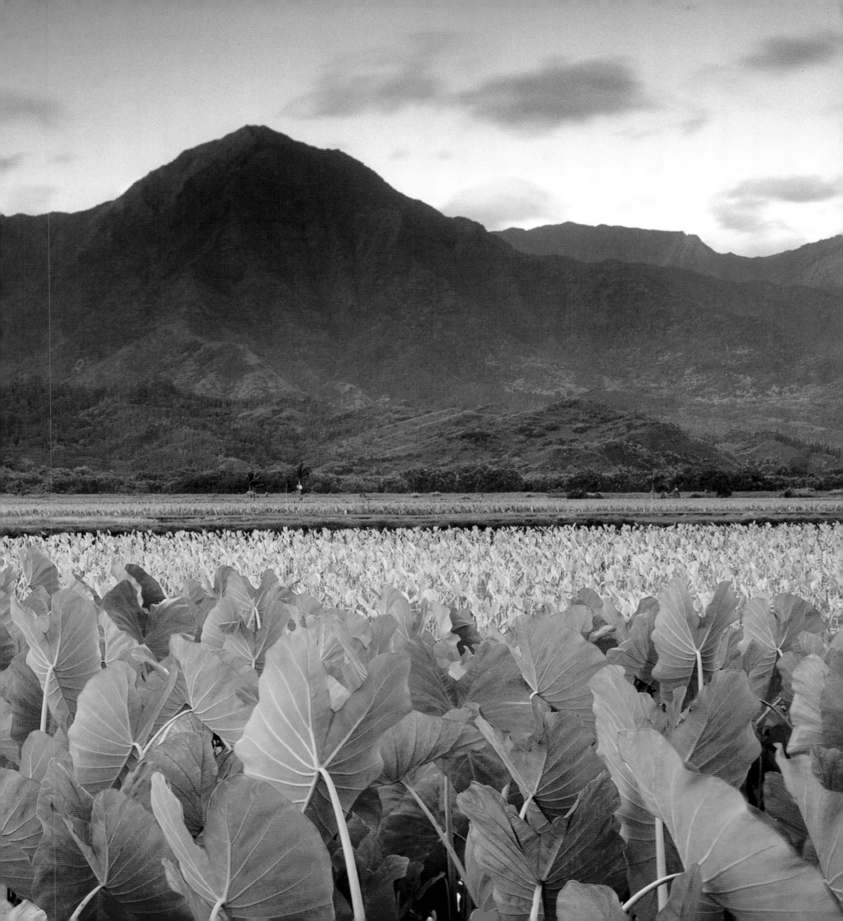

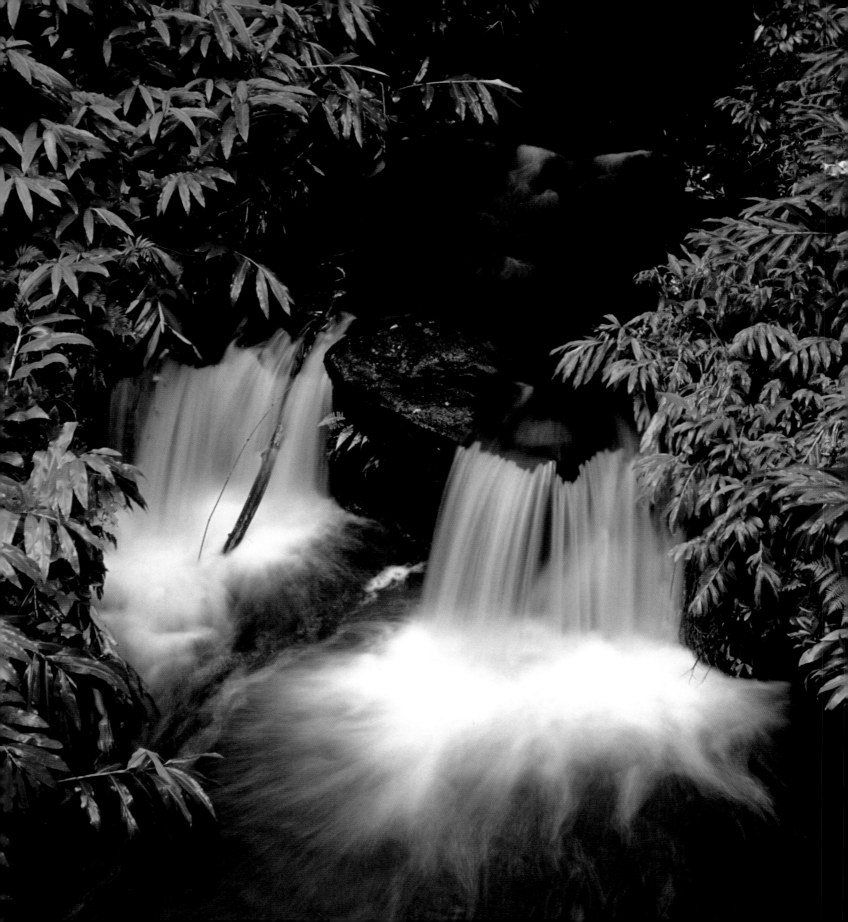

c h a p t e r   1

The ancient Hawaiians recognized that good health begins with good hygiene, and they were meticulous about grooming. They trimmed their hair with implements made of bamboo and shark's teeth, using *kilo pōhaku*, a smooth stone placed underwater in which they could see their reflections. They shampooed with the sudsy sap from the flowers of the fragrant *'awapuhi* (wild ginger), and coaxed tangles from their hair with combs fashioned from the ribs of coconut palm leaves.

After meals, they cleaned their teeth with "floss" (reeds or blades of grass) and "toothpicks" (thin bone or wood splinters). Chewing stalks of sugarcane and rubbing their teeth with a powdered "toothpaste" made from crushed charcoal, salt, or pumice also helped remove plaque and food particles.

The Hawaiians' bathtub was the sea. If they didn't live near the ocean, they bathed in rivers, far downstream from where their drinking water was drawn. They regarded freshwater as the source of *ola* (life), and, as such, they took great care not to pollute rivers, streams, and lakes. After bathing, both men and women perfumed themselves with plants and flowers; the *'ōlena* (turmeric), *maile* (a native twining shrub), and *hīnano* (the male blossom of the pandanus tree) yielded their favorite scents.

Healing involved a holistic approach. When a person became ill, his physical symptoms were seen as manifestations of an inner malaise; thus, the treatment was designed to balance and strengthen his entire being, including his mind, spirit, emotions, and instincts. The Hawaiians understood that outlook greatly influenced overall health; someone who was joyful, loving, forgiving, and at peace with himself and others was more likely to achieve and maintain complete well-being.

PRECEDING SPREAD: As in olden times, taro flourishes in Hanalei Valley, Kaua'i. In addition to being a staple in the early Hawaiians' diet, taro was valued for its medicinal properties.

LEFT: Sitting in cool waterfalls enabled the early Hawaiians to stimulate circulation and ease stiffness.

BELOW: A ti leaf-wrapped *pū'olo* (parcel) rests on the eastern shore of the island of Hawai'i as a gift to the gods.

The *kahuna lapa'au* (medical expert) was highly respected for his extensive knowledge and keen abilities. He did not hold anger or hatred toward anyone, and his intentions were always honorable; a selfish, ambitious, greedy person could not be trusted to wisely exercise the power to heal. Singled out in his village at a young age based on traits such as intelligence, kindness, patience, virtuousness, and a desire to learn, he lived and studied with a master of *'oihana lapa'au* (medical profession), who often was an elder in his immediate or extended family.

His training spanned twenty years, including time in a *heiau ho'ōla* (healing temple) that was dedicated to medical research, the preparation of medicines, and the education of students of *'oihana lapa'au.* He did not

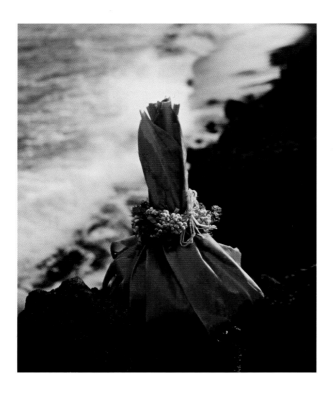

practice without supervision until he had completed his lengthy course of study.

During that period, the student learned by respectfully observing, listening, and imitating his *kumu* (teacher). He didn't ask questions; instead, he pondered and quietly absorbed information with all his senses. Lessons began at dawn and continued as long as there was sunlight. The schedule and curriculum were demanding, but the student worked hard and never complained; he knew it was an honor, privilege, and great responsibility to be one of the few who were chosen to join the *'oihana lapa'au.*

The Hawaiians believed the *akua* (gods) knew all. Worship of the gods was closely linked to the medical arts, and *kāhuna lapa'au* were considered to be the mediums through which the *akua* healed. Prayers and chants formed the foundation of *'oihana lapa'au*, and students spent many hours memorizing and reciting long rituals until they could perform them without error or hesitation. If a practitioner was worthy—if he possessed a pure heart and soul—he would receive the inspiration he needed to diagnose and treat diseases.

In his authoritative book *Ka Po'e Kahiko, The People of Old*, Samuel Kamakau wrote, "If the kahuna was an upright person he would be guided properly by true revelations of his spirit guides; the secret things of his ancestors would be revealed to him, and all the hallowed things about which he did not know. In order to rightly guide the kahuna, and for him to know the proper sacrifices and offerings and suitable prescriptions to use in treatment, he was commanded through akakū (apparitions), hihi'o (visions), kāhoaka (phantoms), huaka (shadowy forms), and 'ike maka (visual knowledge) through seeing and talking with an akua (god) who had assumed human form."

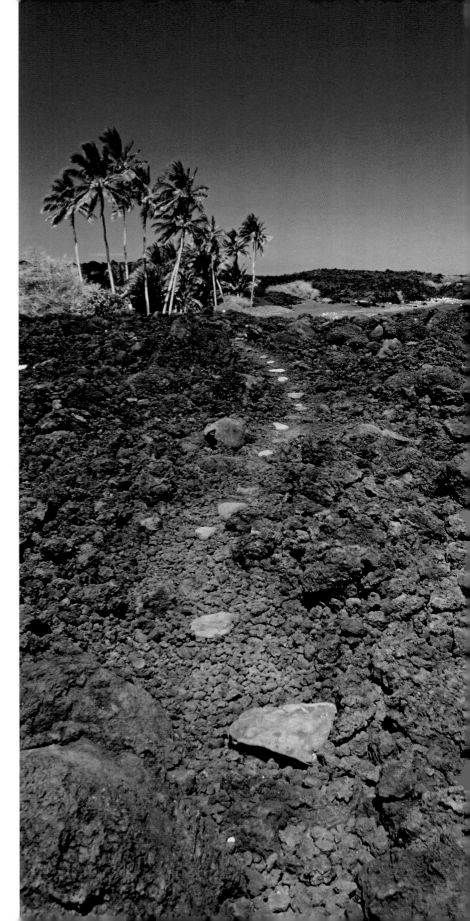

RIGHT: Hawaiians believe all things, including inanimate objects such as rocks, possess *mana* (spiritual power), and are important elements of a balanced and interconnected world.

Kamakau described the general classes of *kahuna lapa'au* as follows:

Kahuna ho'ohāpai keiki and kahuna ho'ohānau keiki:
Who induced pregnancy and delivered babies

Kahuna pā'ao'ao and kahuna 'ea:
Who diagnosed and treated childhood ailments of *'ōmali* (puniness) and *'alalehe* (fretfulness)

Kahuna 'ō'ō:
Who "held back" or kept closed the *ho'opa'a manawa* (fontanel) and practiced lancing

Kahuna hāhā:
Who used a *papa 'ili'ili* (table of pebbles) and the ends of his *wēlau lima* (fingers); that is, who diagnosed by *hāhā* (feel) or palpation

Kahuna a ka 'alawa maka and 'ike lihilihi:
Who could *'alawa maka* (see at a glance) or *'ike lihilihi* (see through the eyelashes) *uwai* (dislocations) and *'anu'u* (sprains), and who diagnosed by insight or critical observation

Kahuna 'anā'anā and kahuna kuni:
Who used *'anā'anā* and *kuni* (black magic) *ma ka lapa'au* (in treatment)

Kahuna ho'opi'opi'o:
Who used *ho'opi'opi'o* (counteracting sorcery) in treatment

Kahuna makani:
Who treated the *makani* (spirits) of illness

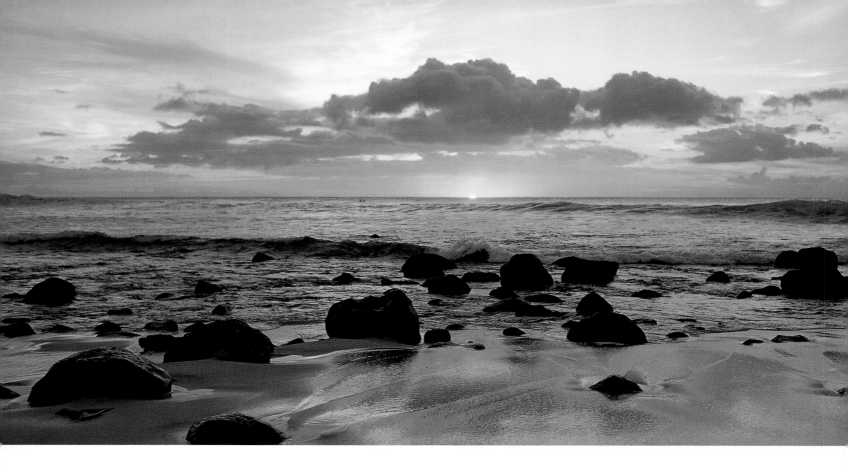

The *kahuna hāhā* could detect physical sickness solely by touch. He learned the art of palpation using the *papa 'ili'ili*—480 red, white, and black pebbles laid out in the shape of a man on a woven mat or piece of tapa. Different arrangements of pebbles corresponded to different disorders. The student deftly worked his fingers over each one, familiarizing himself with the "feel" of the malady it represented. Using this method, he supposedly could diagnose 280 afflictions.

"The study of the pebbles began at the feet," explained Kamakau. "There began the showing of the basic causes of the diseases that men get from the balls of the feet to the crown of the head. There are 100 to 1,000 diseases that snuff out the life of man, and a *kahuna hāhā* must know everything about the body of man."

ANCIENT HEALING PRACTICES

Whenever illness struck, the *kāhuna lapa'au* prescribed a specific course of treatment over a specific span of time. Patients were expected to follow their instructions without deviation. Following is a list of common old-time remedies, some of which are still being practiced today.

'Au'au

Kamakau noted, "For ka po'e kahiko the sea was the remedy upon which all relied." *'Au'au kai* (bathing in the sea) was a common treatment in ancient times. A tilted, chair-shaped stone sometimes can be seen at low tide in Lahaina Harbor, off the west coast of Maui. Long ago, those who were sick sat on this stone, believing the waves would wash over their bodies and cure them.

'Au'au wai (bathing in freshwater) also was therapeutic. Sitting in cool, flowing water, such as in streams and waterfalls, stimulated circulation and eased stiffness. Baths in warm, still water alleviated headaches. Herbs were added to baths to address other problems. For example, *wāwae'iole* (a tropical club moss) was boiled

LEFT: Before it surrenders to night, the sun casts its last rays of light on the vast Pacific along the west coast of Moloka'i. Hawaiian cultural authority Samuel Kamakau observed, "...the sea was the remedy upon which all relied."

in freshwater for about three hours. Bathing in this water when it cooled purportedly helped patients with rheumatism.

The Hawaiians also recognized the restorative powers of sulfur steam vents and warm mineral springs. Scattered along the east coast of the island of Hawai'i are geothermal pools that worked wonders for those with arthritis and muscle pain. Immersion in water, either fresh or salt, often was prescribed as the first and final steps of a regimen.

Food

Food was a vital part of ancient healing traditions. Accompanied by prayers that the patient would recover from his ailment, choice tidbits were among the initial offerings made to the gods and the *kahuna lapa'au*. Before the patient began treatment, feasts sometimes were held for him and his family, with prayers as abundant as the food that was served.

Remedies usually specified which foods the patient could eat and which he should avoid. Fatty meats; raw food; anything seasoned or preserved with salt; and seafood—including squid, mollusks, and certain fish—often were forbidden. So were foods with names that might adversely affect the outcome. For example, *pe'epe'e* means "to hide, camouflage"; therefore, eating the *lipe'epe'e* (a native red seaweed) was not allowed, for it would enable the illness to conceal itself from the treatment. Similarly, *loli* means "to turn, change"; hence, the *loli* (sea cucumber) was excluded from the patient's diet so the effectiveness of the regimen would not be altered.

When the patient had regained his health, there would be a *pani* (literally "to close"), the ritualized preparation and consumption of food that concluded a treatment

and often carried symbolic significance. Just as there was a specific remedy for every disorder, so there was a specific *pani* for every remedy.

One *pani* might consist of *kala* (surgeonfish) or *limu kala* (a common brown seaweed)—appropriate because *kala* means "to release, unburden," and it signified that the person was free of the malady. A *pani* also might include the *lele* variety of banana. *Lele* means "to fly, leap, jump"—another metaphor for sickness leaving the patient. *'A'ama* crab was a third common *pani* food. When captured, the *'a'ama* loses its legs; so does an affliction loosen its grip on a patient when a prescription is successful.

Several everyday foods were valued for their medicinal properties. These included taro (purgative, suppository, stopped bleeding from cuts); sugarcane (sweetened bad-tasting medicines, used as a poultice to heal wounds); guava (for diarrhea, dysentery, sprains, and deep cuts); banana (for constipation, heartburn, listlessness, and chest pains); coconut (for asthma and urine retention); breadfruit (for infected sores and chapped skin); and mountain apple (for thrush, cuts, bronchitis, and sore throat).

Hā

Hā is the breath of life. First, the *kahuna* performed the cleansing *pī kai* by sprinkling or rubbing salt water on the patient's body. Then, as he prayed, he blew *hā* onto the area of concern. His breath activated and directed the *mana* (spiritual power) of the patient to cure the disease, repair bone fractures, or heal whatever was ailing.

The practitioner also might have used *lomilomi* at the same time he was using the ritual of *hā* to guide the healing process. Instead of rubbing or pressing on the

RIGHT: Seawater was mixed with freshwater to make *inu kai*, an effective cathartic.

body, however, he might have used distinctive hand movements to "extract" the cause of the pain, stiffness, or other disability.

In order for the treatment to work, the *kahuna* had to be pure in mind and spirit. He had to be living a righteous life in order to pass love and healing energy through his *hā* to the patient. The patient could feel this energy permeate his body, improving blood circulation, which is a key factor in healing.

Ha'iha'i iwi

Similar to chiropractic, this involved adjusting and setting misaligned and broken bones. Long ago, *ha'iha'i iwi* was used on warriors who had been injured in battle. The *kauka ha'iha'i iwi* (chiropractor) firmly held the patient's shoulders and cracked his bones in a form of joint and spine manipulation that has been compared to modern osteopathic medicine.

Experts of *lua*, a type of hand-to-hand fighting, also were keepers of this knowledge. Bodyguards of the chiefs, these well-trained warriors could break bones, dislocate bones at the joints, and inflict severe pain by pressing on nerve centers. Thus, *ha'iha'i iwi* was used to kill and maim as well as heal.

Hi'uwai

Long ago, this water purification ceremony was held in the latter part of the year, usually November or December. After midnight the people bathed and cavorted in the sea in a rite to wash away the misfortune and adversity of the past year. As dawn approached, they dressed in their finest tapa and ornaments for feasting and games.

For *hi'uwai* today, participants also enter the ocean in early morning, before the first rays of light appear in the sky, to cleanse themselves physically, spiritually, mentally, and emotionally. They emerge from the water with the rising of the sun—symbolically reborn like the new day.

Ho'oponopono

The Hawaiians recognized that *hukihuki* (tension, disagreements) between friends, associates, or family members caused stress, anxiety, fear, and anger that could lead to serious illness. *Ho'oponopono* means "to make right, to bring into proper rhythm and balance." Sometimes lasting an entire day, the session brought together the parties who were at odds in an attempt at reconciliation.

As with *ho'oponopono* practiced today, this involved prayer, discussion, soul-searching, meditation, confession, repentance, apology, forgiveness, restitution, and other means of conflict resolution. Participants let go of grudges and resentment so that peace and harmony could be restored and relationships mended, ideally before the sun set.

Once the air was cleared and the final *pule* (prayer) was uttered, the problem could not ever be brought up again. Wellness starts from within; accordingly, *ho'oponopono* contributed to participants' health by purging the negative feelings and reactions they had to a situation, thus eliminating emotional trauma and internal imbalances.

Inu Kai

One of the most effective cathartics was a concoction of seawater and freshwater. Before drinking it, patients

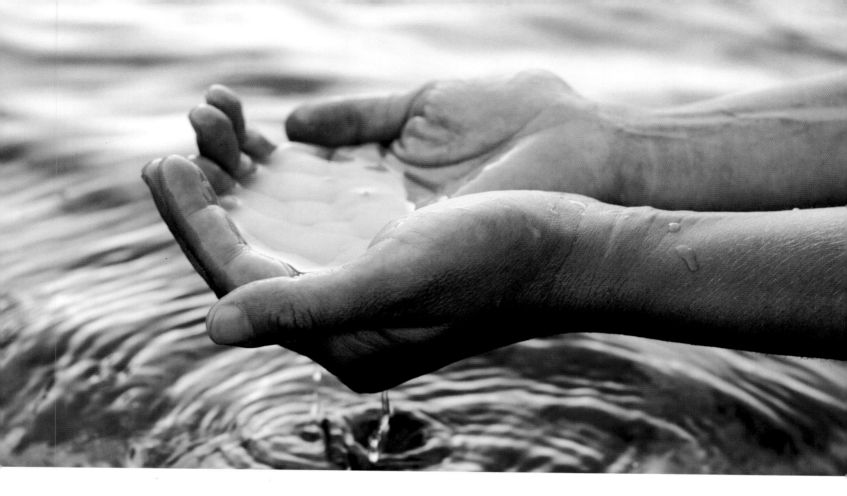

would consume high-fiber foods such as fruits and sweet potatoes to clean out their intestines and bowels. They would then drink the water on an empty stomach.

Kamakau noted, "When people took sick with stomach upsets ('ino'ino ma ka 'ōpū), griping stomach aches (nahu), fever (wela), grayish pallor (hailepo), squeamishness (nānue na 'ōpū), nausea (polouea) [sic], or dizziness (niua) . . . a drink of sea water was the universal remedy employed. . . . They fetched a large container full of sea water, a container of fresh water to wash away the salty taste, and a bunch of sugar cane. They would drink two to four cupfuls of sea water, then a cupful of fresh water, and then chew the sugar cane. The sea water loosened the bowels, and it kept on working until the yellowish and greenish discharges came forth (puka pū no ka lena a me ke pakaiea)." The recipe most often used today is one part of clean seawater to two parts of freshwater.

The Hawaiians also drank freshwater mixed with sea salt and 'alaea (red clay), which is rich in iron. This tonic supposedly strengthened the body's organs and systems.

Kāpaʻi

Herbal poultices were used to treat complaints ranging from bruises, dizziness, and muscle aches to fractures, sprains, and wounds. Plants with antiseptic, anti-inflammatory, and analgesic properties were mashed for application on the skin, usually in the form of a ball or pad. Sometimes a plant was used alone; most often, though, it was pounded into a mixture with salt and other herbs.

Special mortars and pestles were crafted of lava rock to prepare medicinal herbs. Once so designated, they were reserved specifically for this work; they were never used for any other purpose.

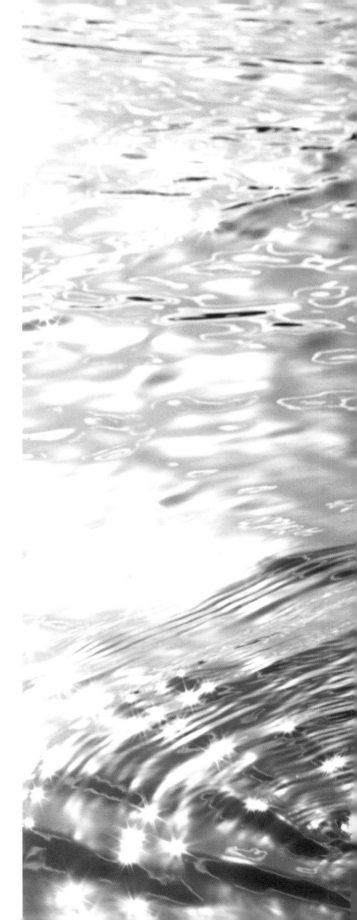

Kapu Kai

Done in privacy, this ceremonial bath in the sea purified those who had come in contact with a corpse or other things considered to be defiled. It also was performed at the end of healing regimens and each time a woman finished a menstrual cycle (she was considered "unclean" during her monthly period). *Kapu kai* was supposedly most effective if it was repeated for five consecutive days.

Sometimes the *kahuna lapa'au* directed a patient to wear a *lei* of *limu kala*, eat some of the plant's seeds and leaf tips, and go swimming in the ocean. *Kala* means "to free, remove." As the patient swam from shore, the waves took the seaweed *lei* from his shoulders and carried it away, thus "releasing" him from his disease.

Lā'au Kāhea

Literally the "calling medicine," this was healing by prayer or speech. In his invocations, the *kahuna lapa'au* requested that his *'aumakua* (family gods) heal the patient. This was done in person, via a proxy, or long distance (that is, with the *kahuna lapa'au* in one place and the recipient in another, perhaps many miles away).

Lā'au kāhea also was used to treat *ma'i 'uhane hele* (spirit sickness)—when the spirit leaves the body and the person is left in a state of depression, with no sense of self or direction. Through *lā'au kāhea*, the *kahuna lapa'au* coaxed the spirit back into the person's body to uplift and motivate him.

Lā'au Lapa'au

The ancient Hawaiians were well versed in the healing properties of plants. Although recipes for common

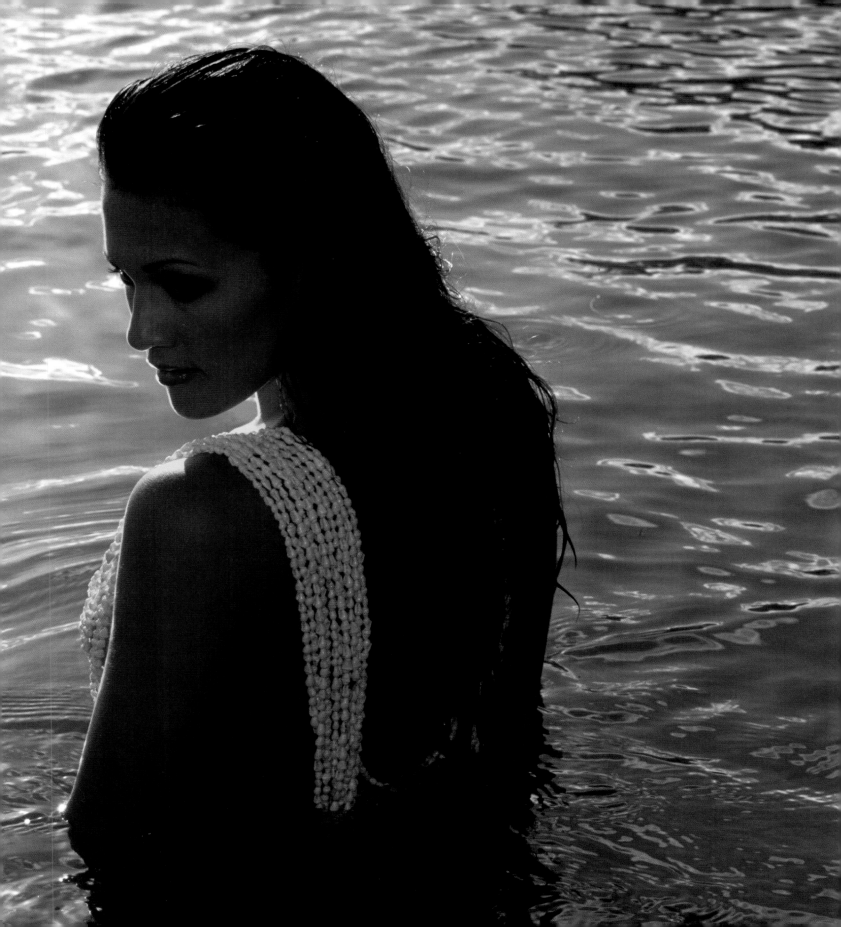

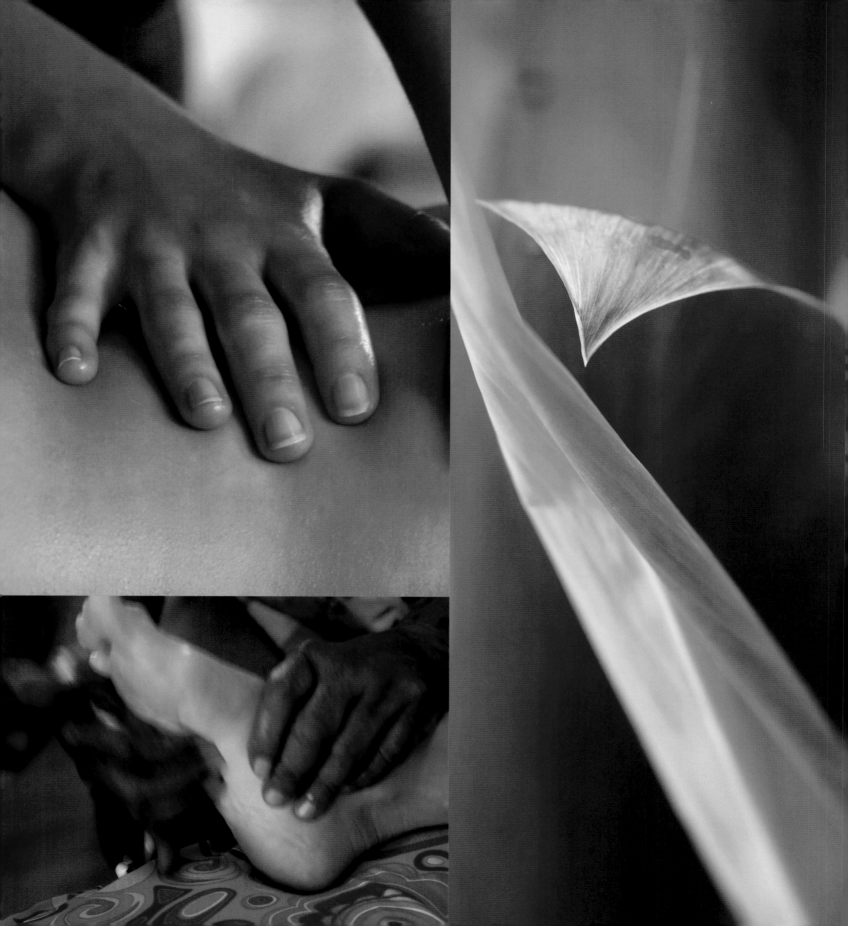

LEFT: The Hawaiians have long recognized the healing powers of plants and the human touch.

disorders often were passed down from generation to generation within the *'ohana* (family), the *kahuna lā'au lapa'au* was regarded as the expert who gathered plants and herbs, and who prescribed, prepared, and administered concoctions made of them.

Botanist, pharmacist, and physician, the *kahuna lā'au lapa'au* learned the names of hundreds of plants, where they grew, what parts were valuable for medicinal use, how they should be prepared, in what proportions they should be mixed, and in what dose and form they should be given. Sometimes his preparations consisted of different parts of the same plant, but more often they were blends of several plants.

Botanical prescriptions were taken internally as teas or extracts, or consumed after being precisely prepared—strained, squeezed, chopped, mashed, roasted, burned, broiled, and/or boiled. They also were applied externally as poultices and dressings. Chapter 2: Nature's Pharmacy contains more information about Hawaiian plant medicine.

Lā'au Nahā

Eliminating wastes from the body either by vomiting or bowel movements was seen as a purification process essential to healing. Seawater, *'akoko* (an endemic shrub), *ipu 'awa'awa* (a variety of gourd), *koali* (morning glory), *kukui* (candlenut), *moa* (a tufted, leafless plant), and *pōpolo* (black nightshade) were common cathartics.

When a laxative was taken orally, abdominal *lomilomi* was performed to help it move through the system. To purge the body, the Hawaiians also used enemas made of bamboo stalks and long, thin gourds.

Lomilomi

Simply defined, *lomilomi* is the art of traditional Hawaiian massage, but in its truest sense, it involves much more than physical touch. Performed by a practitioner with a loving demeanor, clear mind, clean spirit, and pure heart, the bodywork—sometimes gentle, sometimes firm—flushed out negative feelings as well as toxins, resulting in total healing, both inside and out. Prayer is an important part of the process.

In ancient times, *lomilomi* was used to alleviate many maladies, from headache, congestion, and poor circulation to indigestion, edema, and rheumatism. It was performed on women before, during, and after childbirth. It also was used on children to correct birth defects; cure colic and other childhood afflictions; and mold heads, faces, and bodies to desirable shapes.

At once soothing and invigorating, a session might incorporate several different techniques, including rubbing, kneading, squeezing, stretching, bending, rocking, tapping, pushing, pulling, pounding, pinching, and pressing with the hands, forearms, even the feet. Large stones and heavy sticks bent at a forty-five-degree angle also were used to massage, compress, and apply friction to the body.

Lomilomi was not a secret practice; even young children knew how to do it. And, contrary to popular belief, there was no one "correct" technique; masters from different families, villages, *ahupua'a* (land divisions), and islands each had their own unique routines. Even today, there are probably as many different *lomilomi* styles as there are practitioners.

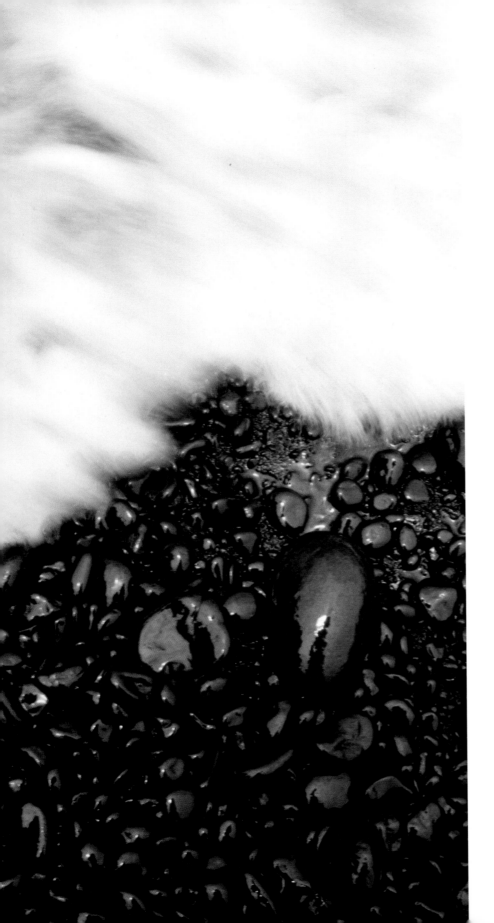

Pī Kai

Performed at the beginning and/or end of a treatment, this ritual involved using a ti leaf to sprinkle the patient, his room, and house with seawater or salted freshwater mixed with 'ōlena root to drive away undesirable spirits that were causing illness. The Hawaiians regarded salt as a cleansing agent and 'ōlena as a powerful force to battle evil. Thus, it was believed the consecrated water of pī kai could remove the dark influences that surrounded a sick person or may have entered his body.

In her book *Hawaiian Herbal Medicine: Kāhuna Lā'au Lapa'au*, June Gutmanis noted, "One prescription advised that a person be naked when he was sprinkled and that the water be poured or sprinkled over the body using a downward motion as in washing. This ritual was followed by a bath and a change to clean or new clothing."

Pōhaku Wela

Hot stones were a common choice for pain and stiffness. Smooth stones were heated in a fire pit, then loosely wrapped in ti or *noni* (Indian mulberry) leaves. The hot packs were placed directly on the patient's problem areas, be it the back, legs, arms, neck, and/or shoulders. The warmth was relaxing and rejuvenating.

The Hawaiians believed all things in nature possessed *mana*, even inanimate stones. They regarded the *pōhaku wela* as conduits that passed energy to "weakened" areas of the patient's body, thus promoting healing.

Pūholoholo

Another effective option for aching muscles and tight joints, this dry sweat bath was done in a *hale hau* (hut

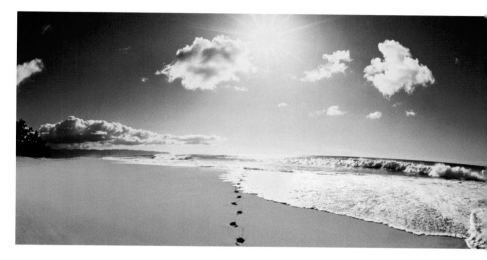

BELOW: Masters of *'oihana lapa'au* prescribed solar therapy for a variety of ailments, including rashes and sore muscles.

made with wood and branches from the *hau*, a low-land tree). The roof arched over an *imu loa* (long oven) filled with stones heated with burning *'uhaloa* and *lama* woods and topped with a thick layer of green leaves (*'ape*, ginger, *koali*, *kukui*, *maile*, *pōhuehue*, *pōpolo*, and ti often were used).

The patient lay on this bed of hot leaves and stones, and was covered with tapa to seal in the heat. When he got too hot, the tapa blanket was removed and his perspiration was wiped off. This was repeated five times.

Pule and Oli

The Hawaiians believed spirituality was the primary aid in healing—more so than any physical therapy. The *kahuna lapa'au* offered prayers throughout the patient's treatment. Likewise, the patient and his family were expected to exhibit faith in the *akua* and to pray often to create an environment that was conducive to healing. If he wanted to get well, the patient also had to have confidence that the prescribed course was going to help.

Oli were sacred chants, invocations to the gods. Remedies for each complaint included the recitation of specific *oli*. The *kahuna lapa'au* was careful to present the *oli* exactly as he had been taught, for even subtle changes in phrasing and pronunciation could jeopardize the efficacy of his efforts.

Pūlo'ulo'u

Good for fevers, colds, chills, and headaches, this steam bath also was done in a *hale hau*. It was important that the house be closed, with no draft. The patient sat on the ground before a large wooden bowl filled with water. Hot stones and herbs were dropped into the bowl, forming steam.

A blanket of tapa or leaves was placed over the patient's head, and he would inhale the steam. This opened clogged nasal passages and drew out impurities through his perspiration. To increase the amount of perspiration, the patient was partially or completely wrapped in tapa, or in ti or *'ape* leaves. Afterward, he cleansed himself in the sea.

Sunning

Mana supposedly is greatest at high noon. For that reason, the Hawaiians regarded the sun as a powerful healing force. Many skin disorders, including rashes and eczema, disappeared after being exposed to direct sunlight. Solar therapy coupled with herbal dressings also was beneficial for fractures, boils, and sore muscles and joints.

One remedy called for swollen tendons to be smeared with the juice of *pōpolo* leaves before exposing them to the sun. Another directed a patient with injured joints to pound *maunaloa* (sea bean) seeds, moisten them with water, and place them in tapa. He then sat in the sun at noon while he rubbed the tapa over the area of his body that hurt.

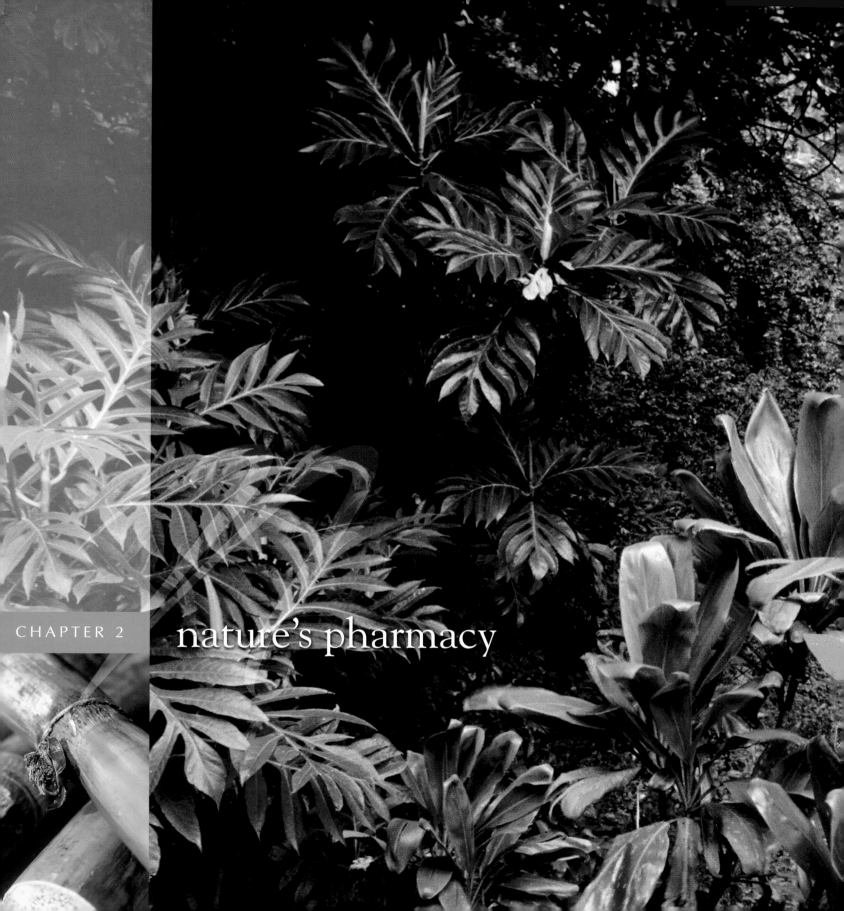

nature's pharmacy

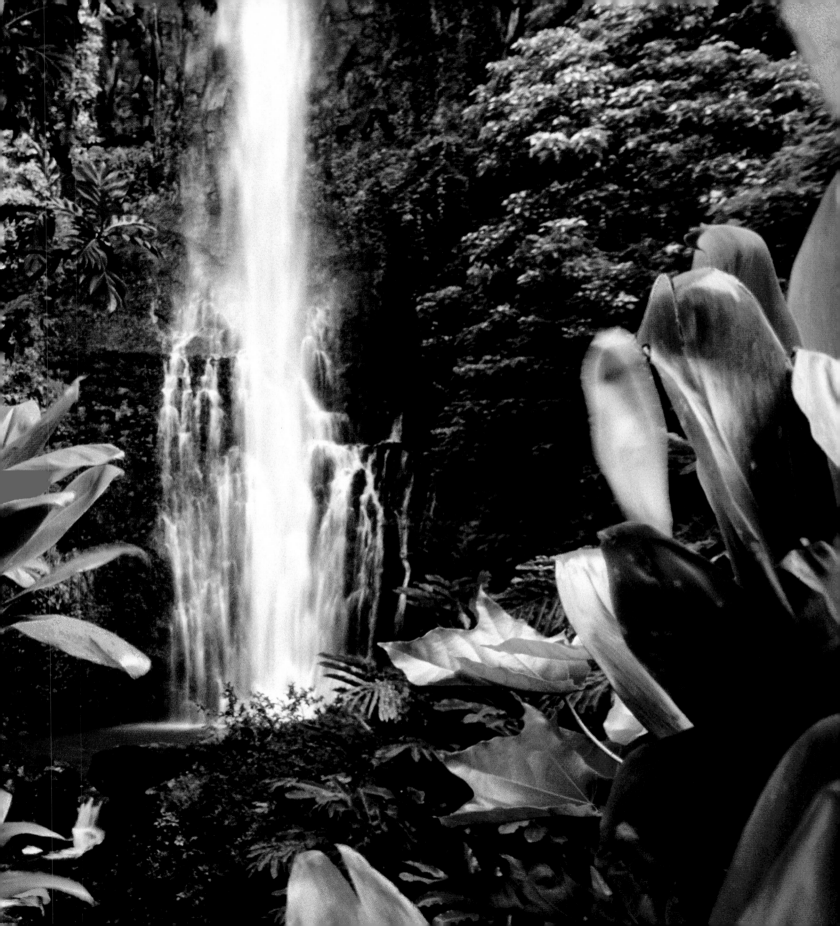

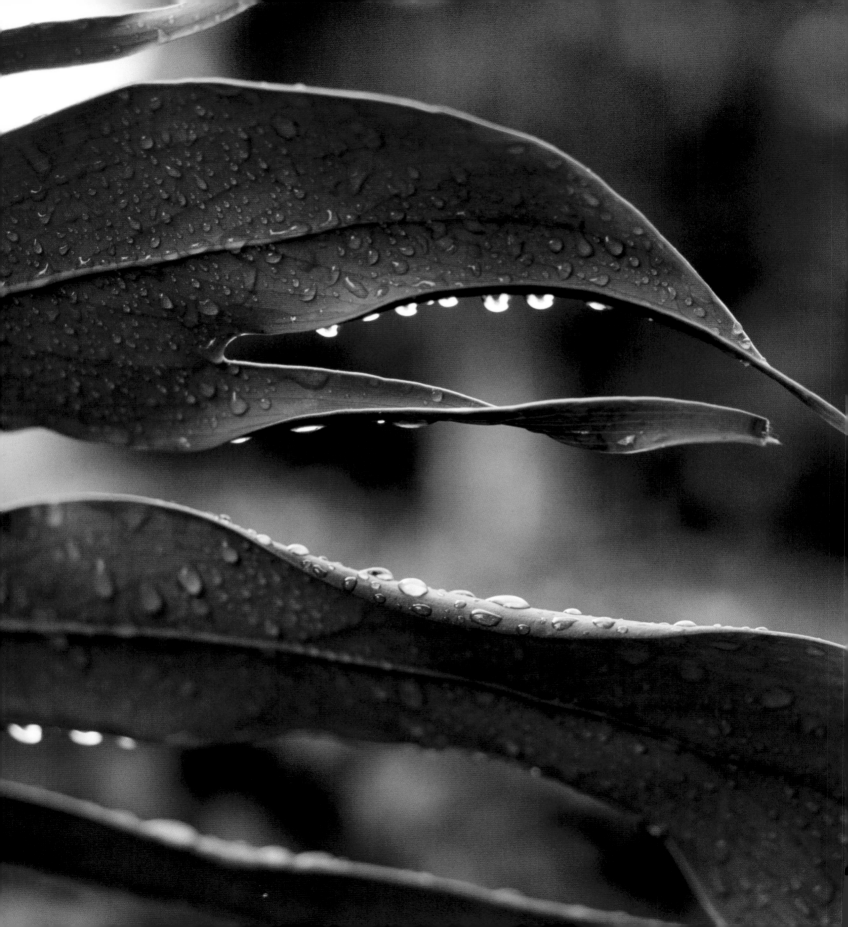

chapter 2

When adventurers from the Marquesas made their incredible voyages across the Pacific to Hawai'i more than fifteen hundred years ago, they carried with them twenty-nine plants that had been carefully chosen for their usefulness. The majority of these plants were food sources. Others were valued because they provided materials for clothing, shelter, canoes, implements, and medicine.

Those resourceful pioneers augmented their pharmacopoeia with native plants and trees that they found growing in great abundance in the Hawaiian Islands' forests, valleys, and coastal regions. Flowers, fruits, leaves, seeds, stalks, stems, sap, juice, roots, even bark were blended in their healing concoctions.

Most of the Hawaiians' traditional medicines were mixtures incorporating ingredients from as many as ten different plants as well as water, pa'akai (salt), and 'alaea (red clay), the latter two known for their effectiveness as

astringents, counterirritants, and prophylactics. Preparations ran the gamut, from mashing fruit and scraping stalks to extracting juice from roots and burning leaves into ashes.

If an internal medication required just one plant, it usually was administered as a tea brewed with wai puna (fresh springwater). Depending on the complaint, recipes specified other types of water—wai pa'akai (salt water); pāhihi (dripping water); wai hī (water trickling from a precipice); wai lani (rainwater); and wai 'apo, wai hua, and wai pū'olo (water caught in taro leaves, deemed pure because it had not touched the ground).

Herbal compounds also sometimes included sea urchins, marine snails, lobsters, hawksbill turtle shells, wood ashes, pālolo (whitish gray clay), 'ana (pumice), and 'elekū (coarse vesicular basalt). Ingredients and

PRECEDING SPREAD: Wailua Falls cascades eighty feet into a pool bordered by tropical greenery in this idyllic vignette of Hāna, Maui.

LEFT: Long ago, nature provided the Hawaiians with the ingredients they needed for medicinal teas, poultices, salves, and more.

doses were measured with halved coconut shells, 'opihi (limpet) shells, and other units that Westerners would consider imprecise; traditional recipes called for items such as "a full handful of flowers," "a piece of bark that will fit in the palm of one hand," and "salt that could be held between thumb and forefinger."

Interestingly, five was the number that appeared most often in prescriptions. The *kahuna lapa'au* (healer) might direct a patient with consumption to drink five portions of a *noni* (Indian mulberry) potion in five days. He might tell a person with back problems to bind five taro leaves on the painful area for five nights before he went to sleep. One cure for constipation consisted of five raw and five cooked *kukui* (candlenuts) mixed with water. To alleviate diarrhea, *pia* (arrowroot) starch was mixed with water and taken five times a day until relief came.

The patient's diet was monitored for the duration of the treatment; for example, the *kahuna lapa'au* might tell him to avoid sour poi and salty foods or to eat a lot of white-meat fish. The treatment concluded with a *pani* (a tidbit of food that was usually, but not always, seafood) and a feast attended by the patient's family.

PLANTS COMMONLY USED IN HAWAIIAN MEDICINE

In a 1934 study entitled *Hawaiian Physical Therapeutics*, noted scholars Dr. E. S. Craighill Handy, Mary Kawena Pukui, and Katherine Livermore listed 317 plants that were used by the early Hawaiians in medicinal treatments, including seaweed, lichens, mosses, and flowering plants. Of these, Dr. Isabella Aiona Abbott (professor emerita, Department of Botany, University of Hawai'i at Mānoa) named the twelve that appear most often in traditional formulas in her authoritative book *Lā'au Hawai'i: Traditional Hawaiian Uses of Plants*: 'awa, 'awapuhi, kalo, kī, kō, koali 'awa, ko'oko'olau, kukui, noni, 'ōhi'a 'ai, pōpolo, and 'uhaloa. Descriptions of these and other significant plants in Hawaiian healing follow.

Research on the efficacy of these plants continues; interestingly, there's no scientific evidence to support the curative powers for the majority of them. Also, details about traditional remedies and many of the requisite prayers that accompanied them have been lost over time, and some plants can be toxic in the wrong doses. In short, be aware that reckless experimentation can be hazardous to your health.

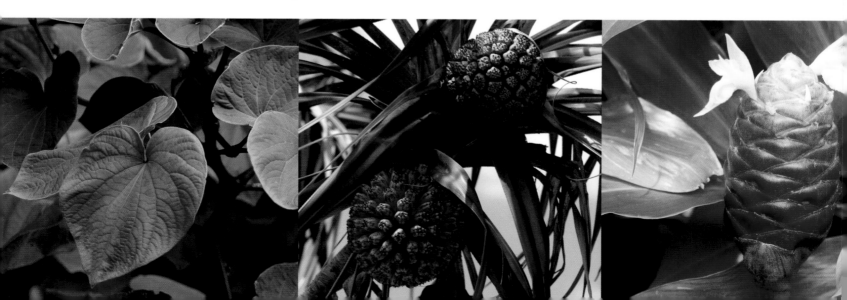

'Ala'ala Wai Nui

Common name: None
Scientific name: *Peperomia* spp.

Parts used: Flower and leaf buds, leaves, sap, stems

Purportedly beneficial for: Asthma, ill-smelling vaginal discharge, infections, infectious diseases, irregular menstrual periods, laryngitis, lower abdominal disease, pulmonary consumption, thrush, uterine abnormalities

Factoid: There are twenty endemic Hawaiian species of this forest herb; ethnobotanists have not been able to determine which ones were used for medicine in ancient times.

'Awa

Common name: Kava
Scientific name: *Piper methysticum*

Parts used: Flower buds, leaves, roots, ashes of roots, shoots, stalks

Purportedly beneficial for: Anxiety, arthritis, chills, difficulty urinating, fatigue, headache, insomnia, kidney disorders, menstrual irregularities, muscle tension and pain, respiratory congestion

Factoid: Drying 'awa brings out its medicinal properties. In fact, fresh undried 'awa is believed to have very little medicinal value.

'Awapuhi Kuahiwi

Common name: Shampoo ginger
Scientific name: *Zingiber zerumbet*

Parts used: Ashes of leaves, flower buds, rhizomes

Purportedly beneficial for: Achy joints, bruises, cuts, dizziness, headache, ringworm, sores, sprains, toothache

Factoid: Its common name refers to the ancient Hawaiians' use of the fragrant sap from its flowering stalks as a shampoo.

Hala

Common name: Screw pine
Scientific name: *Pandanus tectorius*

Parts used: Drupes or wedge-shaped fruitlets, flowers, juice and tips of aerial roots

Purportedly beneficial for: Chest pain, constipation, difficult childbirth. Also used as a cathartic and tonic.

Factoid: Long ago, the leaves were woven into mats, baskets, bedding, canoe sails, fans, and many other utilitarian items. Old drupes with their fibers exposed made excellent brushes to paint designs on tapa.

Hau

Common name: None
Scientific name: *Hibiscus tiliaceus*

Parts used: Slimy sap from stems, flower buds, and inner bark

Purportedly beneficial for: Chest congestion, constipation, dry throat, labor pain. Also used as an enema and internal lubricant to facilitate birth.

Factoid: Dry *hau* wood is very light, sturdy, and buoyant, making it an excellent choice for the outriggers of canoes.

Kalo

Common name: Taro
Scientific name: *Colocasia esculenta*

Parts used: Corms, raw scrapings of corms, sap from stems

Purportedly beneficial for: Constipation (peeled and washed corms cut into cylinders served as suppositories). Also used as a cathartic and to stop bleeding from cuts.

Factoid: To be edible, taro must be cooked; this breaks down the needle-shaped crystals of calcium oxalate in its cells. If it is eaten raw, the walls of the cells burst and the calcium oxalate crystals are rapidly released. They adhere to the lining of the mouth and tongue, causing irritation.

Kauna'oa

Common name: Native dodder
Scientific name: *Cuscuta sandwichiana*

Parts used: Entire plant of yellowish orange thread-like stems and small flowers (it doesn't have leaves)

Purportedly beneficial for: Chest congestion, gangrene, skin infections. Also consumed by women after childbirth to discharge the placenta and blood.

Factoid: Its suction cups attach to other plants, from which it obtains nutrients. Its genus name, *Cuscuta*, is derived from the Arabic word *kusku*, meaning "tangled twist of hair"—an accurate description of the plant.

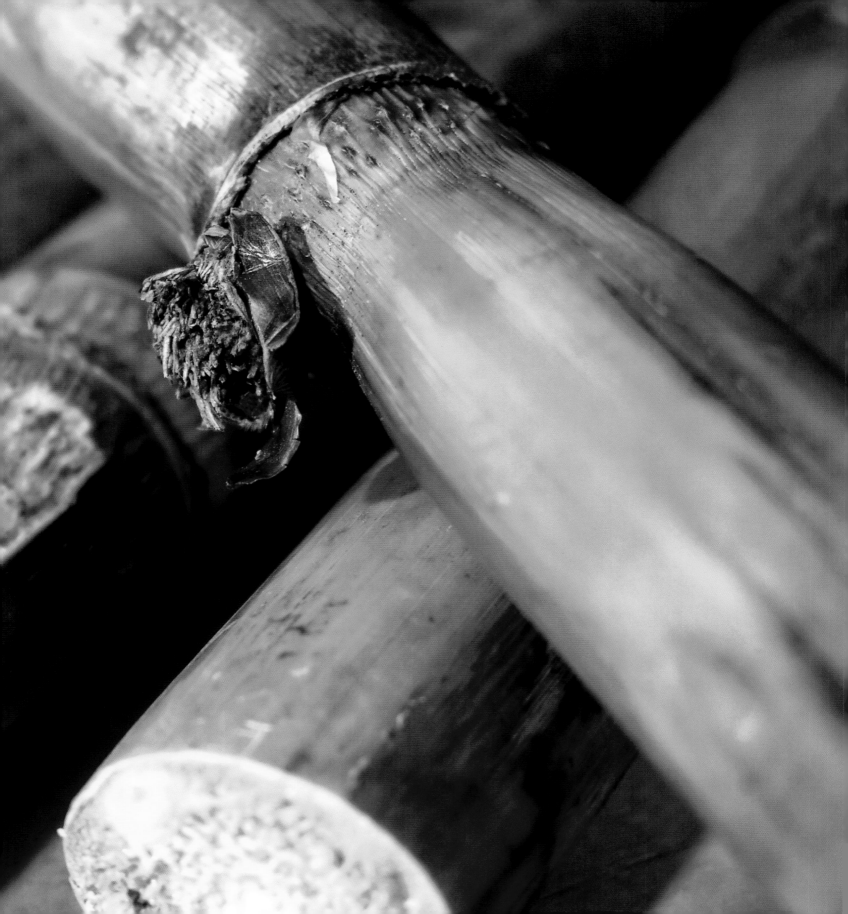

LEFT: Children chewed raw sugarcane stalks to strengthen their gums.

Kī

Common name: Ti
Scientific name: *Cordyline fruticosa*

Parts used: Flowers, leaves, leaf buds, rhizomes, roots

Purportedly beneficial for: Asthma, backache, dry fever, growths in the nose, headache, tuberculosis, vaginal discharge. The leaves were used as compresses and poultices, and were wrapped around heated stones as hot packs.

Factoid: Ti was grown in abundance around houses to ward off evil and bring good fortune. Its leaves had numerous uses in olden times, including whistles, rain capes, sandals, a wrapping for *pū'olo* (parcels), and thatch for houses.

Kō

Common name: Sugarcane
Scientific name: *Saccharum officinarum*

Part used: Leaf buds

Purportedly beneficial for: Cuts, fractured limbs, wounds

Factoid: Sugarcane juice was mixed with bitter medicines to make them more palatable. To strengthen their gums, children chewed pieces of peeled raw stalks.

Koali 'Awa

Common name: Morning glory
Scientific name: *Ipomoea indica*

Parts used: Bark and juice of roots, buds, flowers, leaves, stems, vines

Purportedly beneficial for: Broken bones, constipation, sores, thrush, wounds. Also used as a cathartic.

Factoid: A member of the sweet potato family, this vine often grows more than fifteen feet long. Strong older vines were twisted into rope.

Ko'oko'olau

Common name: Beggar's-ticks, beggar's-lice, Spanish needle
Scientific name: *Bidens* spp.

Parts used: Flowers, leaf buds, leaves

Purportedly beneficial for: Asthma, constipation, throat and stomach problems, thrush, tuberculosis. Also used as a general tonic.

Factoid: *Ko'oko'olau* is the Hawaiian name for the nineteen endemic species in the genus *Bidens*. They are closely related to the common weed beggar's-ticks (*Bidens pilosa*), which was introduced to Hawai'i from the Americas. The Hawaiians recognized the plants' similarities and began substituting beggar's-ticks for the native species in their medicinal concoctions.

Kuawa

Common name: Guava
Scientific name: *Psidium guajava*

Parts used: Fruit, leaf buds, leaves, taproots of young plants, bark of older plants

Purportedly beneficial for: Cuts; diarrhea; dysentery; sprains; joint, tendon, and muscle aches

Factoid: Its wood yields a high-quality charcoal. Guavas have more vitamin C than oranges.

Kūkaepua'a

Common name: Itchy crabgrass
Scientific name: *Digitaria setigera*

Parts used: Leaves, juice and pulp of leaves, shoots

Purportedly beneficial for: Cataracts, cuts, hemorrhoids, infections, infectious diseases, intestinal and stomach disorders, thrush, toothache, ulcers, vomiting blood

Factoid: Regarded as a sacred plant form of the pig demigod Kama-pua'a, it can grow up to forty inches tall.

Kukui

Common name: Candlenut
Scientific name: *Aleurites moluccana*

Parts used: Bark, flowers, leaves, nuts

Purportedly beneficial for: Abscesses, bruises, constipation, sores, swelling, general malaise. Also used as a cathartic and mouthwash.

Factoid: It is Hawai'i's state tree. About 80 percent of the nut is oil. Centuries ago, whole nuts were strung together and lit as candles, hence its common name "candlenut" tree.

Laukahi

Common name: Broad-leaved plantain
Scientific name: *Plantago major*

Part used: Leaves

Purportedly beneficial for: Boils, diabetes, high blood pressure, kidney problems, thrush, *wana* (sea urchin) spine wounds

Factoid: Scholars believe it was brought to Hawai'i by early Chinese immigrants. The Hawaiians gave it the same name as their native *laukahi* and began using it as a medicinal herb.

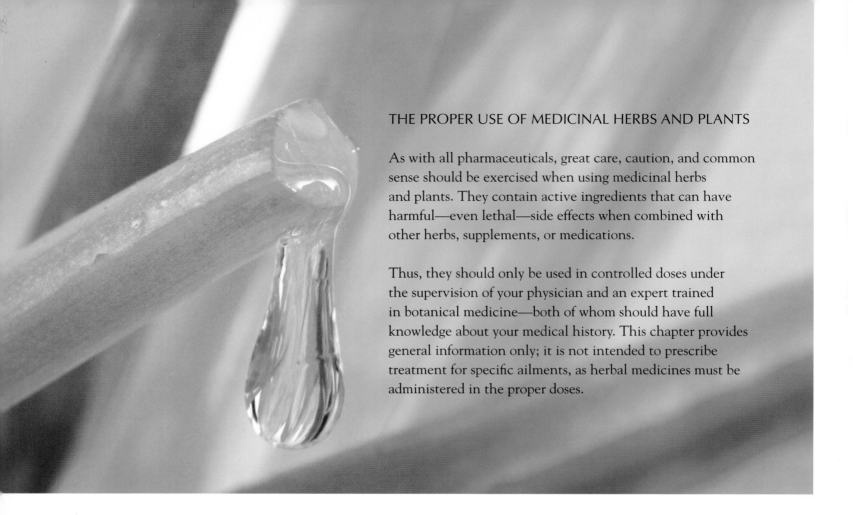

THE PROPER USE OF MEDICINAL HERBS AND PLANTS

As with all pharmaceuticals, great care, caution, and common sense should be exercised when using medicinal herbs and plants. They contain active ingredients that can have harmful—even lethal—side effects when combined with other herbs, supplements, or medications.

Thus, they should only be used in controlled doses under the supervision of your physician and an expert trained in botanical medicine—both of whom should have full knowledge about your medical history. This chapter provides general information only; it is not intended to prescribe treatment for specific ailments, as herbal medicines must be administered in the proper doses.

Noni

Common name: Indian mulberry
Scientific name: *Morinda citrifolia*

Parts used: Leaves, bark of stems, fruit, juice

Purportedly beneficial for: Boils, bruises, compound fractures, constipation, cuts, diabetes, high blood pressure, kidney problems, skin infections, sores, wounds. Also used as a tonic.

Factoid: The red substance in the inner bark of the trunk and the yellow substance in the inner bark of the root were used as dyes in ancient Hawai'i. Although it's not very tasty, the mature fruit is edible and was eaten in times of famine. It is a member of the coffee family.

'Ōhi'a 'ai

Common name: Mountain apple
Scientific name: *Syzygium malaccense*

Parts used: Leaves, juice from bark and branches

Purportedly beneficial for: Bronchitis, cuts, halitosis, sore throat, thrush, wounds

Factoid: Eating large amounts of the fresh fruit causes diarrhea—something that doesn't occur if you dry the fruit before eating it.

'Ōlena

Common name: Turmeric
Scientific name: *Curcuma longa*

Part used: Rhizomes

Purportedly beneficial for: Cough, earache, sinus problems, sore throat, stuffy nose

Factoid: The ancient Hawaiians used it in purification ceremonies, and its roots were a source of yellow dye for tapa. 'Ōlena is a member of the ginger family and is an ingredient of mustard and curry powder.

Pānini 'Awa'awa

Common name: Aloe
Scientific name: *Aloe barbadensis*

Part used: Clear jellylike mucilage from inner portion of leaves

Purportedly beneficial for: Blisters, burns, lacerations, minor skin irritations, wounds

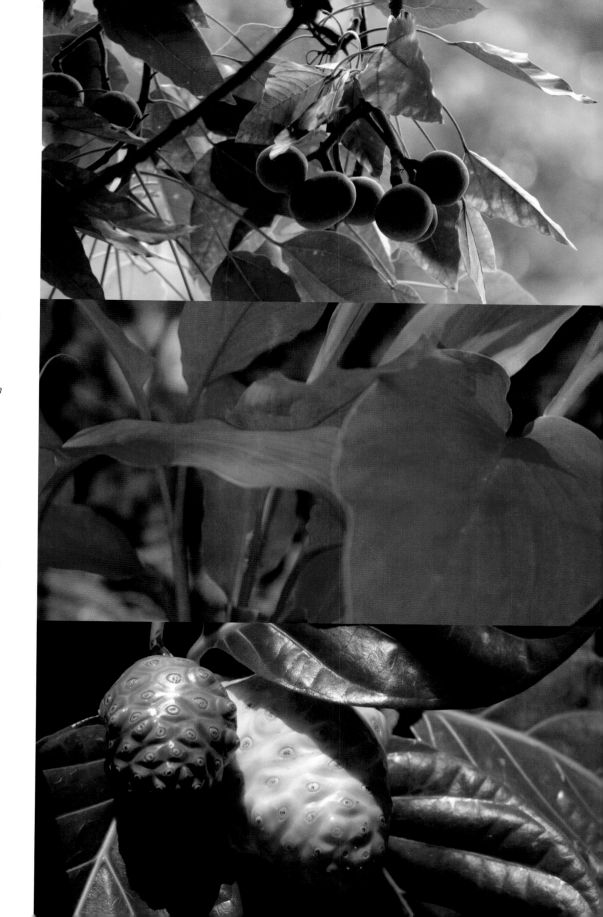

Factoid: There are more than 250
species of aloe, which, despite its
cactus-like appearance, is a member
of the lily family. It ranges in size from
one inch to two feet in diameter.

Pōpolo

Common name: Glossy nightshade
Scientific name: *Solanum americanum*

Parts used: Bark of taproots, leaves,
juice from leaves and ripe berries

Purportedly beneficial for: Asthma,
abdominal trouble, cuts, respiratory
disorders, skin problems, wounds.
Also used to strengthen the immune
system and build red blood cells.

Factoid: Among the most important
of the Hawaiian medicinal plants, it
was believed to be one of the physical
forms assumed by Kāne—the creator of
man, the great god of all living things.

'Uhaloa

Common name: Waltheria
Scientific name: *Waltheria indica*

Parts used: Bark and juice of taproots,
flowers, leaf buds, leaves, stems

Purportedly beneficial for: Asthma,
cough, sore throat. Also used as a
tonic.

Factoid: Quite hardy, it grows in dry
areas from sea level to four thousand
feet in elevation on all of the main
Hawaiian Islands. The sap from its
taproot has the pain-relieving benefits
of aspirin.

Remedies

The following remedies are from June Gutmanis's book *Hawaiian Herbal Medicine: Kāhuna Lā'au Lapa'au*. They are to be considered as general guidelines only, taking into account her admonition "that most are only fragments of more complex prescriptions. In all cases, they would have originally included an opening, the instructions for the gathering of the ingredients, the central herbal prescription which is the part most generally given here, the *pani* (or closing food), and a feast of thanksgiving. At every step there would have been prayers, and no medicine would have been administered without first having put things 'right' with the gods and man."

Cold

For colds resulting in a run-down condition, boil the bark of the mountain apple tree slowly and thoroughly. Drink some before eating.

Constipation

To compound an effective enema, pound together five raw and five cooked *kukui* nuts, add hot water, mix, and strain. When cool, administer.

Earache

Pound *'ōlena*, put it into a cloth, warm it, and squeeze it into the ear.

Headache

Pick several young, tender *ki* (ti) leaves. Remove the middle rib and stalk, dip in cold water, wipe dry, and tie around your head. Remove as soon as the leaf is warm and dry. Replace until your headache is gone.

High Blood Pressure

Take the very ripe fruit of the *noni* and mash. Drink the juice, when eating, for five days. Repeat until cured.

Insect Stings

For a sting from an insect, cut the stem of any kind of taro and rub over the afflicted part.

Insomnia

When it is difficult to sleep, or when suffering from pain, drink a large potion of *'awa*.

Sprains

Cut the top of a very young sugarcane shoot. Mash it up, putting in plenty of Hawaiian salt. Wrap it in ti leaves. Cook over a charcoal fire. When ready, squeeze the juice into a container, saturate a cloth, and rub over the injured area.

Wounds, Cuts, and Sores

For cuts and skin sores, mix ashes of the *'awapuhi* with ashes of the small leaf bamboo and juice from four green *kukui* nuts. Apply to the sore spot.

FOOD AS MEDICINE

Four hundred years before the birth of Christ, the Greek physician Hippocrates advised, "Let food be your medicine and let medicine be your food." Revered as the Father of Medicine because many of his practices are still used by doctors today, he made note of more than three hundred herbs, spices, fruits, vegetables, and other nutritional substances that he believed played key roles in the healing process.

It was Hippocrates who introduced the notions that rest, fresh air, diet, and exercise have a profound effect on physical and mental well-being, and that plants provide a cure—or at least notable relief—for many ailments.

Take a good look around your kitchen. You may be surprised to find how many natural pharmaceuticals you regularly stock in your cupboard and refrigerator.

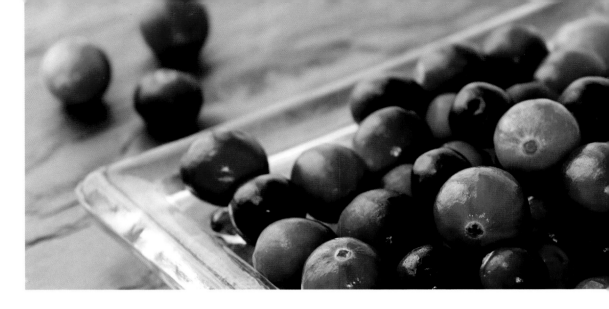

RIGHT: Cranberries contain proanthocyanidins (PACs), which inhibit bacteria from adhering to the urinary tract, thus preventing infection.

Alfalfa

Scientific name: *Medicago sativa*

Parts used: Flowers, leaves, sprouts

Purportedly beneficial for: Diabetes, high cholesterol, infections, menopause, menstrual discomfort

Cautions: Don't use alfalfa if you have systemic lupus erythematosus or other autoimmune diseases. It can cause diarrhea and stomach upset.

Blueberry

Scientific name: *Vaccinium* spp.

Parts used: Fruit, juice or extract, leaves, stems

Purportedly beneficial for: Diabetes, diarrhea, viruses, intestinal inflammation. Also supposedly can improve vision.

Cautions: None

Clove

Scientific name: *Syzygium aromaticum*

Parts used: Flower buds and oil

Purportedly beneficial for: Digestive problems, gum disease, halitosis, mouth pain, sore throat, toothache

Cautions: During pregnancy, it should be safe to use clove as a food spice, but don't use it medicinally. The oil may cause skin and mouth irritations.

Cranberry

Scientific name: *Vaccinium macrocarpon*

Part used: Ripe berries

Purportedly beneficial for: Kidney stones, urinary tract infections

Cautions: None

Dandelion

Scientific name: *Taraxacum officinale*

Parts used: Leaves, roots

Purportedly beneficial for: Bloating, dyspepsia, edema, gas, liver disorders, loss of appetite. It also purifies the blood.

Cautions: It should be used with care if you have obstruction of the bile ducts and/or gallbladder, ulcers, gastritis, gallstones, or gallbladder disease. It can cause dermatitis and dehydration.

Fennel

Scientific name: *Foeniculum vulgare*

Parts used: Leaves, seeds

Purportedly beneficial for: Abdominal pain, digestive problems, gas, halitosis, menstrual disorders. It also increases the production of milk in lactating women.

Cautions: Don't use fennel if you have a chronic disease of the gastrointestinal tract such as stomach or duodenal ulcers, reflux esophagitis, or colitis. It can cause uterine contractions in pregnant women. The oil can cause nausea, vomiting, rash, and seizures.

Garlic

Scientific name: *Allium sativum*

Part used: Bulbs

Purportedly beneficial for: Colds, earache, fungal skin infections, high blood pressure, high cholesterol, intestinal parasites, respiratory infections

Cautions: Don't use garlic if you're nursing, taking a blood-thinning drug, or about to undergo a surgical procedure, as it can cause postsurgical bleeding. It can cause heartburn, flatulence, and gastrointestinal upset if five or more cloves are consumed daily. It also can cause skin irritation.

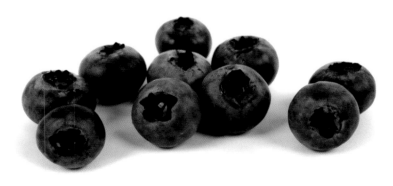

Ginger
Scientific name: *Zingiber officinale*

Part used: Rhizomes

Purportedly beneficial for: Fever, indigestion, morning sickness, motion sickness, muscle aches, rheumatoid arthritis, vomiting

Cautions: Don't use ginger if you're at risk for miscarriage or have gallstones or a chronic disease of the gastrointestinal tract such as stomach or duodenal ulcers, reflux esophagitis, or colitis. It can cause diarrhea, heartburn, and vomiting.

Papaya
Scientific name: *Carica papaya*

Parts used: Fruit, inner bark, leaves, seeds, stems

Purportedly beneficial for: Constipation, indigestion, insect stings, intestinal parasites, snakebites, sores, warts, wounds

Cautions: Don't use papaya if you're taking a blood-thinning drug or if you have gastritis, ulcers, or reflux esophagitis. It can cause uterine bleeding, heartburn, and skin irritations.

Parsley
Scientific name: *Petroselinum crispum* and *Petroselinum sativum*

Parts used: Leaves, roots, seeds, stems

Purportedly beneficial for: Edema, gas, halitosis, indigestion, kidney problems, menstrual disorders, urinary tract infections

Cautions: Don't use parsley if you're pregnant or if you have an inflammatory kidney condition. It can cause dehydration, dizziness, nausea, and photosensitivity.

Peppermint
Scientific name: *Mentha x piperita*

Parts used: Leaves, oil

Purportedly beneficial for: Flatulence, colic, indigestion, irritable bowel syndrome, nausea, painful menses, stomach cramps

Cautions: Don't use peppermint if you have gallstones, ulcers, or liver or gallbladder disease. The oil can cause esophageal reflux, heartburn, and mouth irritations.

Red Raspberry
Scientific name: *Rubus idaeus*

Parts used: Fruit, leaves

Purportedly beneficial for: Childbirth, diarrhea, heavy menses, intestinal inflammation, mouth irritations, sore throat, tonsillitis

Cautions: It can cause diarrhea and nausea.

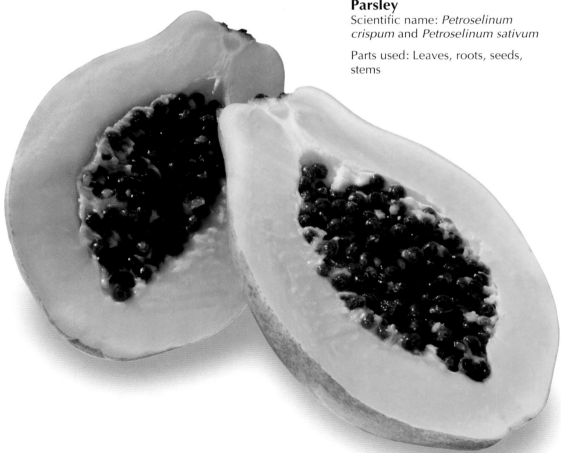

Rosemary

Scientific name: *Rosmarinus officinalis*

Parts used: Berries, fruit, flowers, leaves

Purportedly beneficial for: Depression, halitosis, headache, indigestion, joint pain, memory loss, sore muscles

Cautions: It can cause diarrhea, nausea, skin irritations, and vomiting.

Sage

Scientific name: *Salvia officinalis*

Part used: Leaves

Purportedly beneficial for: Depression, fever, indigestion, mouth irritations, profuse perspiration, tonsillitis, wounds

Cautions: It can cause dry mouth, swelling of the lips, and uterine contractions in pregnant women.

Thyme

Scientific name: *Thymus vulgaris*

Parts used: Flowers, leaves

Purportedly beneficial for: Asthma, bronchitis, cough, digestive problems, fever, fungal and parasitic infections, throat infections

Cautions: Don't use thyme if you're pregnant, as it can induce menstrual discharge. The oil can cause dizziness, headache, nausea, sweating, and vomiting.

THE RUNDOWN ON HERBS

These tips will help you properly select, store, and prepare your herbal ingredients.

Educate yourself so you're able to recognize and obtain the best quality of herbs available. The effectiveness of your remedies is directly related to the quality of herbs you use to make them. Whenever possible, buy organic herbs or those that have been grown in the wild—or, better yet, grow your own. Most are hardy and will thrive even in limited space and in less-than-ideal soil conditions.

You can determine quality herbs by their color (should be vivid, bright, deep, and "alive"); scent (should be strong and distinctive, but, remember, not all herbs have pleasant smells); taste (should be fresh and pronounced, although not all herbs taste good); and effectiveness (should produce the therapeutic results you seek).

Fresh herbs are preferable to dried herbs. If fresh herbs aren't available, dried herbs can be used, but be aware they should retain pretty much the same color as when they're fresh.

Store dried herbs in glass jars with tight-fitting lids. Affix a label to the jar that specifies the name of the item; the date you obtained it; and instructions for use (the recipes for which it's an ingredient, contraindications, whether it's for internal or external use, and any other comments). Keep accurate records; mistakes could result in concoctions that are harmful to your health.

Avoid storing your herbs in areas exposed to light, heat, or air, as these elements will quickly destroy their flavor and potency. Insects and age also are enemies of herbs. Stored in a cool, dark kitchen cabinet or pantry, herbs should last several months or even years.

These are the common kitchen tools you'll need to prepare herbal concoctions—pots, pans, bowls, strainers, large spoons, graters, cheesecloth, coffee grinder, measuring cups and spoons, and glass bottles and jars.

Important: Don't use aluminum or copper containers or tools, as both metals will react with and diminish the quality of herbs. Instead, opt for cookware made of glass, stainless steel, ceramic, cast iron, or enamel.

Remedies

Cranberry Broth

1   c. cranberries
2   c. water
Honey to taste
1   Tbsp. potato starch
2   Tbsp. cold water

Heat cranberries and water until cranberry skins open. Strain out berries and add honey. Heat mixture again to just below boiling, then remove from stove. In a separate bowl, mix potato starch with cold water. Slowly add this mixture to the cranberry juice. Blend well. Return mixture to heat and bring to a full boil, stirring until it thickens and becomes slightly transparent. Cool. Put in a covered container and store in refrigerator until ready to use. It alleviates the symptoms of colds and is a good source of vitamins B and C.

Three Seed Tonic

1   tsp. whole fennel seeds
1   tsp. whole fenugreek seeds
1½ tsp. whole flaxseeds
3   c. water
Lemon to taste

Simmer seeds in water for 15 minutes. Strain out seeds, add lemon, and drink. It eases constipation, upset stomach, gas, and coughs.

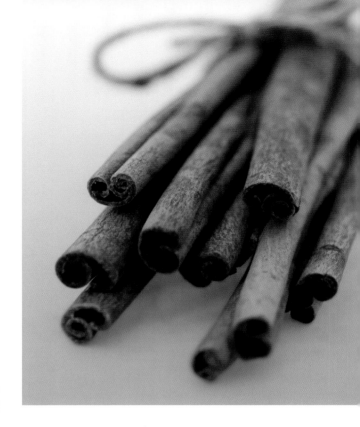

Cinnamon Clove Throat Soother

2   Tbsp. bruised whole cloves
2-3 cinnamon sticks
Pinch bruised whole caraway seeds
2   c. inexpensive sherry

Steep ingredients and store in a bottle in a dark closet. Shake often. After 1 to 2 weeks, strain out herbs. Add 1 teaspoon to 1 tablespoon of mixture to a glass of water for use as a gargle for sore throat.

Parsley-Raspberry Cold Remedy

1   tsp. fresh or dried parsley leaves
2   raspberry leaf tea bags
1   c. boiling water

Steep parsley and tea bags in water for 5 to 10 minutes. Strain out parsley and drink. Take 2 or 3 times a day to clear mucus and congestion during the first stage of a cold or flu.

LEFT: Cinnamon adds flavor to a homemade gargle (see recipe below photo).

Honey Lemon Cough Syrup

½   c. honey
¼   c. lemon juice
¼   c. whiskey

Put all ingredients in a jar and mix well. To quiet a cough, take 1 or 2 teaspoons every 4 hours either alone or mixed in a cup of hot water or tea with a few slivers of fresh ginger.

Garlic Earache Treatment

1   clove fresh garlic, peeled and sliced
1   Tbsp. olive oil

Heat garlic and olive oil for 1 minute. Strain out garlic. Put a few drops of warm garlic oil extract into affected ear and seal with a ball of cotton. Lie down for 15 minutes with affected ear facing up, then rise and tip your head to allow excess liquid to drain out.

Headache, Be Gone

• Roast a handful of caraway seeds. Put them in a soft handkerchief or piece of muslin, tie the ends to make a pouch, and sniff.

• Crush 10 to 15 holy basil leaves (tulsi), 5 or 6 peppercorns, and a half-inch slice of fresh ginger into a powder. Store in an airtight bottle. When needed, mix 2 pinches of the powder in a cup of warm water and drink it.

• Remove the skin and the core of a ripe apple. Cut the apple into slices, sprinkle them with a little salt, and eat them on an empty stomach.

• Boil a handful of rosemary in 4¼ cups of water. Pour liquid into a bowl. Cover your head with a towel and inhale the steam for as long as you can. Repeat until your headache has dissipated.

Tackling Toothache

• Chew a clove or a piece of ginger with the aching tooth to draw out the juice. Let the clove or ginger rest on the tooth for 30 minutes. Repeat 2 or 3 times.

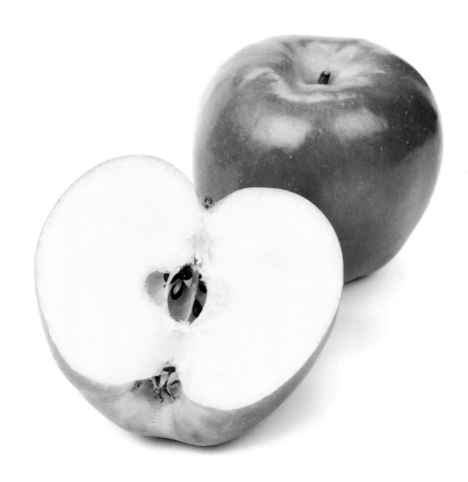

• Boil 2 tablespoons of salt or 1 teaspoon of peppermint and a pinch of salt in 1 cup of water. Let the liquid sit until it's lukewarm, then rinse a mouthful of it around the sore tooth.

• Peel and crush a clove of garlic, mix it with a little salt or peanut butter, and apply it to the painful area.

• Chew a piece of raw onion with the affected tooth for 3 minutes or place the onion directly on the tooth.

Peppermint Cooler

1 qt. purified water
⅓ c. fresh or dried peppermint leaves
Ice cubes

Boil water, then pour over peppermint leaves. Cover and steep for 10 minutes. Strain out leaves and cool mixture to lukewarm. Add ice cubes to chill it (or put in freezer). Soak a cloth in the concoction and wring until it doesn't drip but retains enough liquid to stay cold. Apply for fever, burns, blisters, or insect bites or stings. When the cloth gets warm, soak it in the chilled liquid again and reapply. Repeat 3 to 5 times, adding ice cubes if necessary. Thoroughly dry the area after treatment is complete.

Thyme for Yourself Tea

2 tsp. dried thyme
2 tsp. dried spearmint
2 tsp. dried sage
6 c. boiling water
Honey to taste

Using a tea ball or mesh tea infuser, put herbs in a teapot and pour water over them. Steep for no more than 10 minutes. Pour tea immediately into cups and serve with honey. A few cups a day will relieve menstrual cramps and the tension and moodiness that often accompany PMS. This tea also is good for coughs, fever, colds, flus, and stomach problems. A stronger tea is effective as a mouthwash or rinse to treat sore gums.

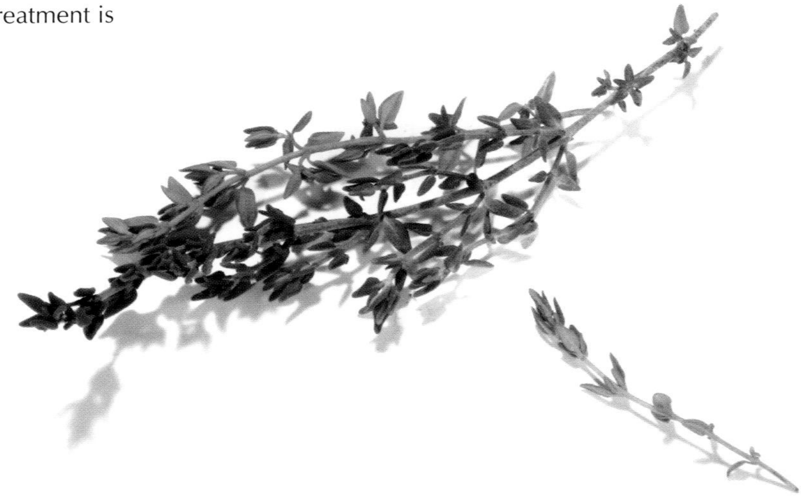

BELOW: Herbal teas have been touted worldwide for their medicinal properties.

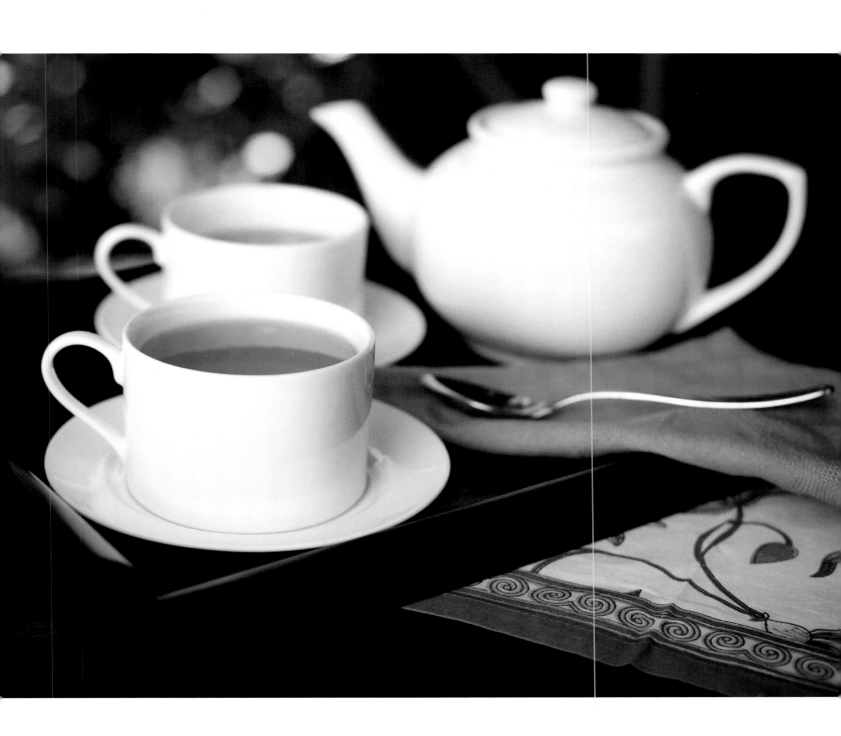

sharing aloha: the gift of healing

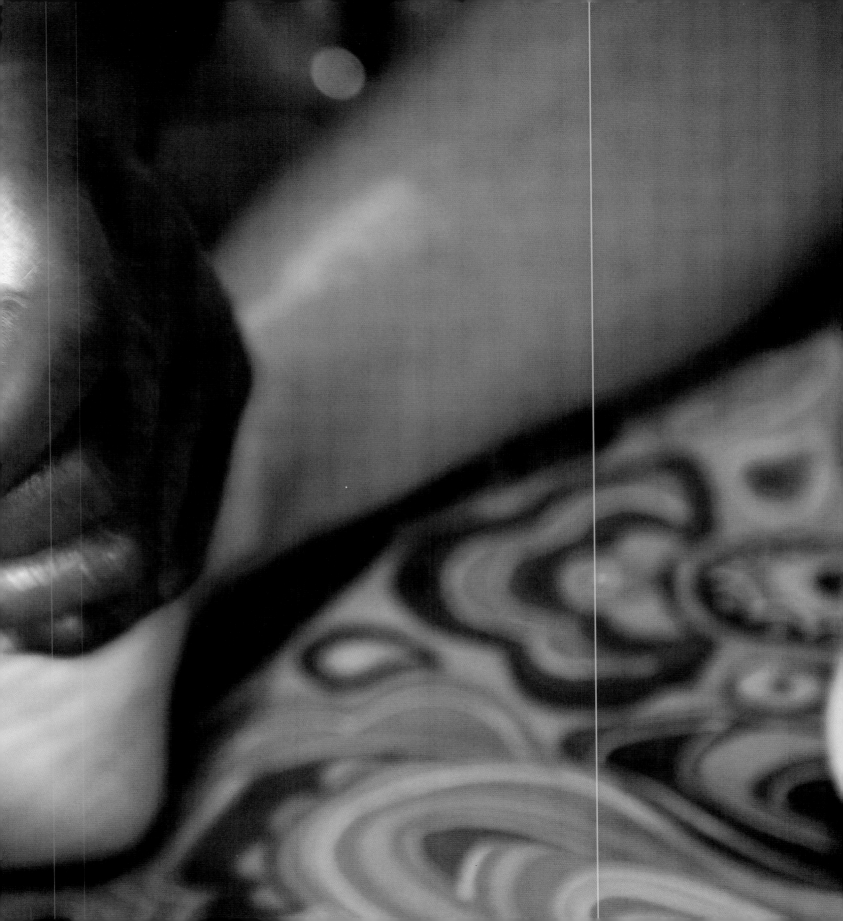

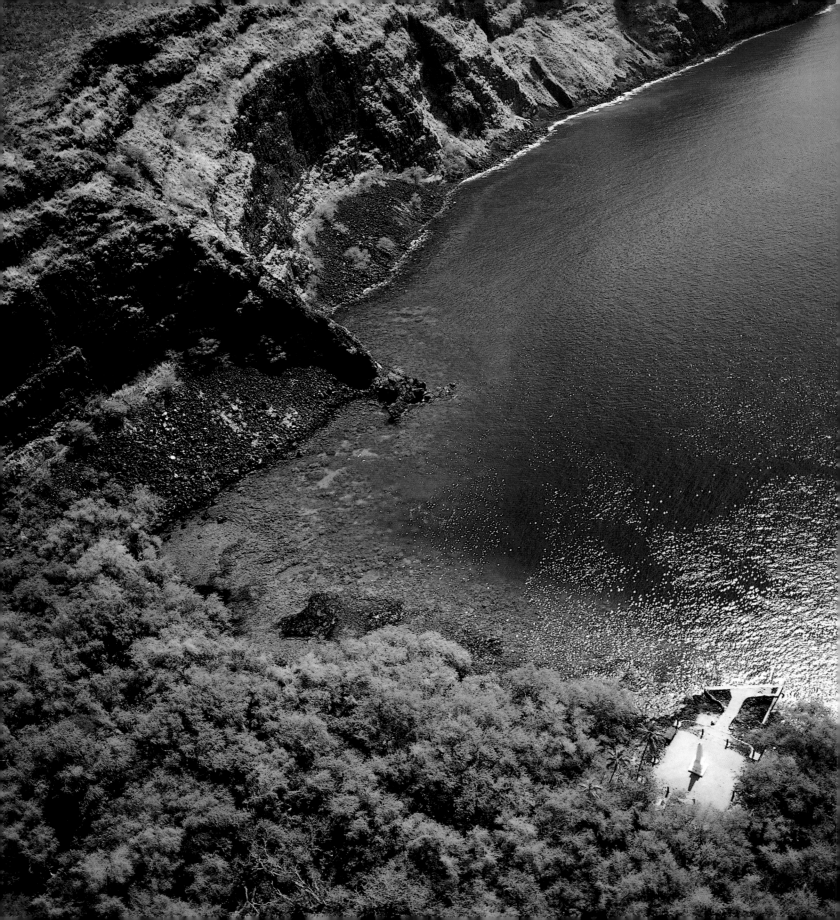

c h a p t e r   3

W hen British Captain James Cook opened Hawai'i to the Western world in 1778, the Hawaiians' traditional way of life began to quickly disappear. The foreigners brought new religion, language, food, attire, customs, and medicinal practices—essentially a whole new way of life—to the islands.

They also brought diseases to which the Hawaiians had no immunity. Many *kāhuna lapa'au* died before they could impart all their knowledge to students. The rest went underground, their methods of cure discouraged by Christian missionaries, who were becoming a major influence in island society. New medicine men with university degrees and stethoscopes took their place.

For decades, *'oihana lapa'au* remained submerged, practiced primarily by families in the privacy of their homes. Only in recent years has there been a resurgence of interest in and acceptance of traditional Hawaiian healing arts.

From a cultural standpoint, this is heartening, but, unfortunately, much of what the ancient healers knew has been lost; in many cases only fragments of prescriptions have been preserved and passed down through the generations. Also, people with questionable pedigrees have come forth, claiming to be "experts" in everything from *lomilomi* to herbal medicine. How can you distinguish a true expert from a charlatan? One way is to determine his credentials. Ask what his "lineage" is; that is, ask who was his teacher, his teacher's teacher, and so on.

Another method of discernment is to evaluate his works, not his words. An old Hawaiian saying goes: *'Ike 'ia nō ka loea i ke kuahu,* which means, "An expert is recognized by the altar he builds"—it is what one does and how well he does it that shows whether he is an expert or not. Following are profiles of twelve esteemed Hawaiian cultural practitioners who are ably carrying on the work of their ancestors.

PRECEDING SPREAD: Sylvester Kepilino deftly performs *lomilomi* on a patient's foot. To be successful in this work, practitioners must have a pure heart, clear mind, and loving demeanor.

LEFT: A white stone monument beside Kealakekua Bay, island of Hawai'i, honors Captain James Cook, who is credited with discovering the Hawaiian Islands in 1778. The subsequent influx of foreigners affected every aspect of the Hawaiians' way of life, including their medicinal practices.

Mary Fragas
Hilo, Island of Hawai'i

In September 1929, Mary Fragas, then six years old, attended her first day at Honoka'a High and Grammar School. The next day she was stricken with polio, which left her paralyzed from the neck down. Back then, doctors didn't know much about polio, and she was left in the care of her parents. Every day until Fragas was able to return to school at the age of thirteen, her mother and father took turns massaging her to keep her warm. Her parents massaged her with no thought, no knowledge, that doing so would help her get better, but Fragas, the oldest of eleven children, believes their efforts saved her life. Besides her, twenty-three other children at the school contracted polio. Several years later, she heard all of them had died.

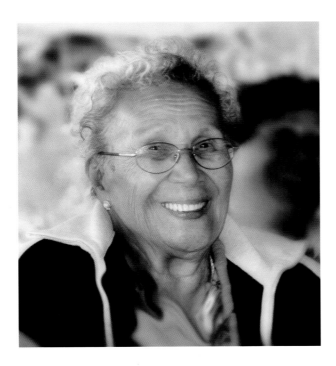

I went to sleep at night wondering why my classmates had died and why I was still alive. Then click: the thought came to me about Mom and Dad massaging me. They had unknowingly kept me alive by massaging me and increasing my circulation. They never failed to massage me day and night, night and day. They didn't know it at the time, but warmth was the answer.

Still, I wasn't "cured." I can't say I have really ever been able to walk normally. I force myself to walk by throwing my right shoulder forward and the right leg follows. I throw my left shoulder forward and my left leg follows. That's how I've been able to move about. It's the same thing with my arms and hands. Sometimes I use a cane or crutches. But if my parents didn't massage me, I know I would have been bedridden or probably dead by now.

Regarding learning *lomilomi*, my parents never taught me; they never said, "You do this and you do that." I just watched what they were doing when they massaged me. Years later, as an adult, I became interested in *lomilomi* when I realized that it could help other people, not only me. I asked experts if it would be okay for me to watch what they were doing. I also read books on anatomy. That's how I learned.

Today, people with all kinds of problems come to see me, and somehow by watching them walk and looking at them as they're lying on my mat on the floor, I am able to figure out what is wrong with them. I can tell just by looking; thoughts appear in my mind, telling me what to do with patients. I can feel where their pain is and where I'm supposed to work. I know this ability is a gift. This is what I'm supposed to do—help people.

Lomilomi consists of stroking, pressing, and kneading. There isn't just one correct method of *lomilomi*; there are many ways to do it. But the Hawaiians massage on the floor; you can give pressure more effectively if the patient is lying on the floor. In ancient times, the Hawaiians never had tables. They worked on a *lau hala* mat on the floor.

There is no set time frame for my treatments. I work on my patients for a while, then I ask them to turn over and I continue massaging them until I feel it's sufficient. When they get up and walk around, the majority of them feel better, more relaxed. And that's what matters.

In the morning, I always pray. I ask God to help me with the work I'll be doing on patients that day. I ask Him to show me how I can help each person who comes to me. Prayer gets me in the right frame of mind and spirit.

I don't ask for money; I never have. Many people can't afford to pay money, but they give me what they can, from their heart. They bring me vegetables, papayas, avocados, fish, *'opihi* [limpets], *poi*, a bag of oranges or grapes—things like that. I can tell they're very grateful by the gifts they bring.

Anybody can do *lomilomi* if they delve in the thought of wanting to help people. We're all born as God's children, we all can help one another. But if you're only going to massage someone because you want money, you're not going to last, that's for sure. You really have to want to help people. That's what makes a true healer.

Kawaikapuokalani Hewett
'Ōla'a (Mountain View), Island of Hawai'i

Kumu hula (hula master), *singer, musician, and author of over one hundred songs and chants (more than any other living Hawaiian composer), Kawaikapuokalani Hewett is regarded as one of the foremost authorities on Hawaiian language and culture. He learned* hula *and the*

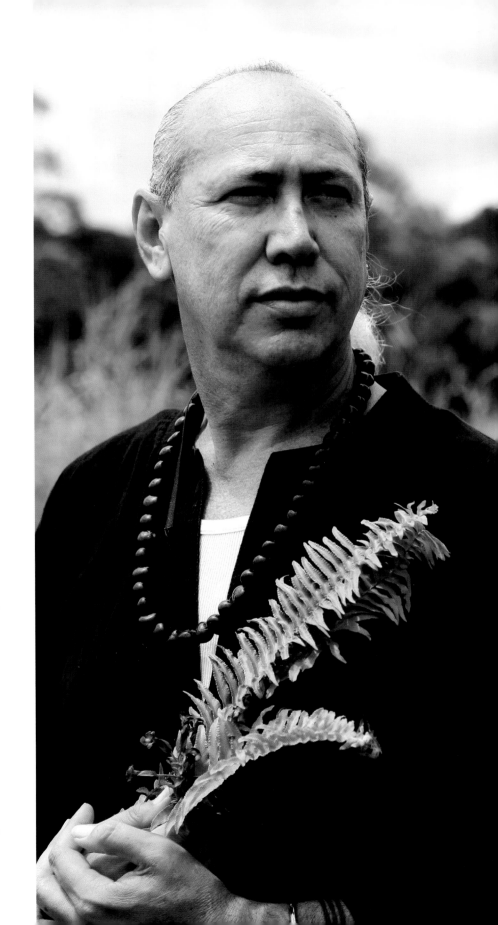

healing arts from his grandmother at an early age, and continued his studies under respected kūpuna *such as Sam Lono, Edith Kanaka'ole, and Emma DeFries. Hewett recently brought his life's dream to fruition—Kahalelehua (the house of the* lehua*),* lehua *being a metaphor for an expert or someone who possesses great skills. Set amid thirty-five acres of lush forest and pastureland on the slopes of Mauna Loa, it is a serene retreat where students come to live and learn* hula *and Hawaiian medicinal practices from* kumu *and* kahuna ho'ōla *(healer) Hewett.*

When I was growing up in Kāne'ohe on O'ahu, it was our family tradition to camp at Ka'a'awa Beach Park. In the summer of 1972, right after I graduated from high school, my family went to Ka'a'awa as usual. When we were setting up our tent, there was a woman in the water with long, flowing white hair. She was dressed in a red *kīkepa* [sarong]. I was told not to go near her because she was a *kahuna,* and I needed to be careful.

For me, that meant the exact opposite; it made me want to meet her even more. So I walked to a spot a short distance from where she was, and she started to talk to me. She told me that she would be my teacher and I would be her legacy. That was how I met Auntie Emma DeFries.

A few days later, Auntie Emma went to see my grandmother and told her she wanted to train me. My grandmother consented, and they changed my name from Frank to Kawaikapuokalani, which means "sacred water of heaven." It was important to change my name to show that I was reborn, in a sense. My new name was to be a protector, a guide, my strength.

And so at eighteen, I was adopted by Auntie Emma to start a new life, to begin my journey in the tradition of healing. I trained with her for nine years. She came to stay at my home, I stayed at her home. She was the care-taker of Queen Emma Summer Palace in Nu'uanu, and she had a little cottage in back of the palace. Most of the time, my training took place at the beach in Ka'a'awa. We would often be there from dawn until dusk.

The beach is symbolic. From a psychological perspective, it is very calming, very soothing. In the Hawaiian culture, it also represents release. Salt water is used to bless, it's used to purify. Every day, as soon as the sun came up, we would be in the water doing our ritual cleansing. That is how our day would start. We also did a ritual bath before the sun set.

My lessons ranged from practical to deep and spiritual. I was drawn to the ancient traditions; they seemed familiar to me. Auntie Emma always remarked how much I knew already, but what I knew was solely from intuition. Healing came second nature to me.

Kuleana, responsibility, is a big part of Hawaiian medicine. The *kahuna* might say to cure a certain condition, you have to exercise, follow a strict diet, and drink herbal teas. Some people will say, "I might as well just take a pill." And that's what they do because taking responsibility for their illness is too much effort.

Prayers and rituals also are essential parts of the Hawaiian way of healing. The healer has to say the right prayers and do the right rituals, which are shared judiciously by knowledgeable teachers. They're very sacred—not something you would just hand over to your neighbor like a cookie recipe. They reflect practitioners' *mana,* their authority to heal.

There are three ways to identify a true Hawaiian healer: outward purity, inward purity, and his or her relationship with God. Such healers need no certificate. If their work is successful, people will continually seek their help.

If their work is not, people will not go to them. Healers should be judged by the same criteria as our ancestors—by the quality and success of our work. Nothing else.

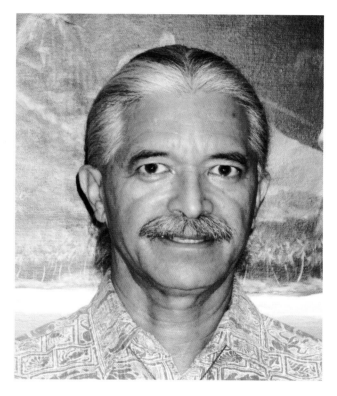

Kai Keali'ikea'ehale O Kaholokai
Kawaihae, Island of Hawai'i

Growing up on O'ahu and the island of Hawai'i, Kai Keali'ikea'ehale O Kaholokai gathered food and medicinal plants from the ocean and mountains for his family's frequent parties. Being an avid outdoorsman, he was always happy to do this, and thus came to know food as medicine, medicine as food. Whenever Kaholokai, his four siblings, or 147 cousins got sick, they would take remedies made by the kūpuna *(elders). They never asked questions; all they knew was if they took the concoctions, they would get well. Kaholokai thought that would be the extent of his involvement with Hawaiian plant medicine, but shortly after graduating from high school he made a lifestyle choice to "go back to the basics." Today he is regarded as one of the foremost messengers on the subject.*

I stopped using Western drugs over thirty years ago when I realized nature provides me with all the medicines I need. I know where these plants grow, so I gather what I need and replant. You could call me a Hawaiian Johnny Appleseed.

Every family has their own medicinal recipes. For instance, my grandma on my mom's side of the family lived in Waimea on the Big Island, so she knew about the mountain and forest plants. My grandpa on my dad's side lived in Waiau on O'ahu, so he was familiar with the plants by the sea that were good for medicine. I was fortunate to be exposed to both.

When I was a teenager, many people I knew were getting sick and dying, and I wanted to stay healthy. I asked my *kūpuna* what I had to do, and they told me about medicinal plants. At the time, though, I was lifeguarding and teaching swimming, and I wanted to surf and travel. I was interested in plants, but I had other priorities.

They sensed that I had a gift and said the time would come when I would realize plant medicine was my calling. I thought, *Yeah, right*, and didn't pay much attention to that. In 1973, I moved from O'ahu to the Big Island and it hit me: *Now is the time for me to focus on the plants.*

I learned from many knowledgeable people—my grandparents, Auntie Margaret Machado, Uncle Tommy Solomon, Papa Kalua Kaiahua, and others. They emphasized the spiritual aspects of healing; that is, they said I had to take care of my inner self as well as my body. I had to have a pure heart, forgive people, set things right.

Healing is about balancing the spirit. Negativity manifests itself physically as "dis-ease." You seek something outside of your body for balance and are told that consumption of this plant or that plant is the answer. But without a strong spiritual relationship with yourself, your god, and nature, you'll only receive temporary relief.

Complete healing is not only about physical consumption; just ingesting plant medicine will not necessarily cure you. Prayer, meditation, and purging negative feelings also are important. If you don't address the mental and emotional concerns that you have, your symptoms may go away for a while when you consume the medicine, but they'll come back. Two people might take the same medicine, and it'll work for one person but not the other, because he didn't have the spiritual element of healing. He first needs to forgive or change his attitude about the person, thing, or situation that's the root of his problem.

In fact, you don't have to consume the plants; you can benefit from their healing power just by being around them. It's like being among great leaders; you don't have to physically touch them to be inspired. Or when you do *lomilomi*, it soothes tense muscles and pain, but you also help the recipient feel safe, protected, and cared for.

Much of the healing process concerns what we can't see. The *kūpuna* will tell you 90 percent of healing relates to the spirit. For me, spirit means knowing my purpose, utilizing my gifts, enjoying being of service, and expressing love, which is aloha.

Alo is being in the presence of the Creator. *Hā* is the breath of life. Sharing *hā* puts us in the presence of the

Creator's love. Aloha touches us on a deep level, awakening our soul and spiritual awareness, and empowering us to take responsibility and action for our own healing and potential for greatness.

Charles Ka'upu
Nāpili, Maui

Charles Ka'upu has taught Hawaiian history, culture, and religion throughout the islands as well as at prestigious mainland organizations such as National Geographic and the Smithsonian Institution's National Museum of the American Indian in Washington, D.C. He is a respected kumu hula *who's known for his expertise in* oli *(chants). Before the arrival of the Christian missionaries in 1820, the Hawaiians had no written language. All knowledge—including their genealogy, legends, family stories, medicinal recipes, and reports of important events—was passed orally from generation to generation. Chants and prayers asking for blessings, inspiration, and* kōkua *(help) from the* kūpuna *and* 'aumakua *(family or personal god) also figured prominently in ancient healing rituals. Ka'upu has shared, utilized, and experienced the power of this spiritual communication many times in his life.*

In order to heal whatever ailment you might have, body, mind, and spirit all are important. You must first acknowledge that you are in control and can overcome the sickness or injury. One of the most important things in the healing process is a positive frame of mind.

And you must do whatever is required for the body to get better, whether it be putting on the salve or drinking the herbal concoction. The spiritual element links to the mind because you have to believe that the treatment will work. You have to have faith that it will help you and you'll get better. This is where chants and prayers come into play. Unlike Western medicine, where only drugs usually are used to heal a condition, the Hawaiian way is holistic, incorporating all these elements for healing to take place.

I had no formal training in Hawaiian medicine; it became automatic to me because it was part of my daily life at home. It was ingrained in me because I remember my parents, my grandparents, and others in their generations doing it.

When we kids had a cold or sore throat, we were told to chew on the root of the 'uhaloa [waltheria]. It's really bitter, and you have to eat sugarcane or orange slices afterward to take the ugliness from your mouth, but you do get well. If we were constipated, we would eat about a teaspoon of baked kukui nuts and that would solve the problem. If we had thrush, the sap from green kukui nuts would be rubbed in our mouths, which induced vomiting. Basically, kukui nuts purge the body.

Plant medicine has worked for thousands of years. It's real. You know the plants the medicines came from, as opposed to Western medicine, where many drugs have been synthetically produced.

There wasn't only one prescription for each ailment. Families had their own recipes, and not every plant and animal could be used by everyone. For example, if your 'aumakua was the shark, then you wouldn't eat it. If your 'aumakua was a certain kind of fish, you wouldn't eat that either. Some animals have corresponding plant forms, so those plants also would be off-limits to you. Out of respect, you wouldn't ingest them in any way, shape, or form, for they are the things that protect you. Long ago, it even went so far that if a fish that was kapu [taboo] to you was roasting on an open fire and you walked through the smoke or inhaled it, you would get sick and possibly die.

In ancient times, the kāhuna were the PhDs of society. Kahuna means priest or expert in any profession. No ifs, ands, or buts—they were the specialists and they knew their craft inside and out. Usually, medicinal knowledge was passed down within a kahuna family, but sometimes the kahuna chose to tutor someone outside his family if he saw that person possessed a special gift for healing.

That decision is never questioned; kāhuna who deal in the spiritual realm are given insight that other people don't have. And just because you're born into a kahuna

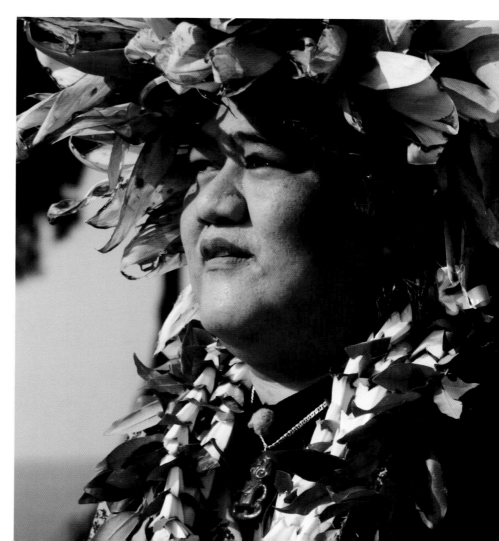

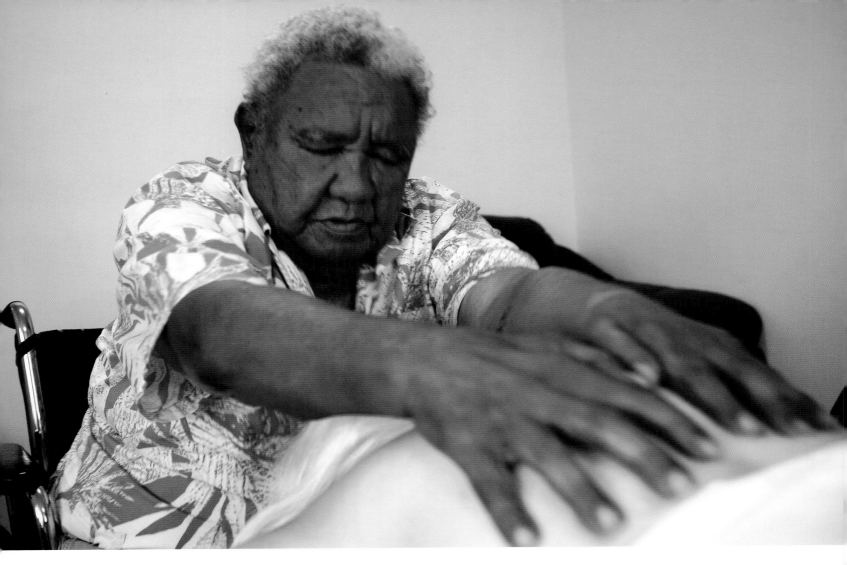

family doesn't mean that you're a *kahuna*. It simply means that you come from that line.

The word *kahuna* is being used too loosely today. How can you determine who's a real *kahuna*? It's called *hana lima*. Do. Acknowledgment comes by doing. You don't need to toot your horn and say, "Look everybody, I'm a *kahuna*," because your works, what you do, will determine whether or not you're worthy of calling yourself a *kahuna*.

Sylvester Kepilino
Hilo, Island of Hawai'i

Sylvester Kepilino, affectionately known as "Papa K," traces his lineage back to the great warrior king, Kame-hameha I. He comes from a distinguished line of Hawai-ian healers that includes both of his parents and his paternal grandfather, who raised him. Although he has no written records to confirm it, Kepilino believes there were many other healers among his progenitors, because in ancient times knowledge about the healing arts was kept within the same 'ohana (family). It was carefully guarded—it usually was not shared with outsiders—and when the time came to name a successor, it typically was the eldest son. There were fourteen children in Kepilino's 'ohana—*seven boys and seven girls. Breaking tradition, his grandfather surprisingly chose him, the youngest child, instead of his oldest brother, to carry on the work.*

One afternoon when I was six years old, my grandfather said to me, "Come, Tutu." That was my nickname when I was small. I said, "Where are we going?" He said, "We're going to take a walk in the forest."

Grandpa took me up into the mountains in Ho'okena and started building a lean-to out of *hāpu'u* ferns. He told me to pick *liliko'i* [passion fruit], *pohā* [cape gooseberry] and *'ōhelo* [a native shrub in the cranberry family] berries, and the white inner stems of the ti plant.

As I was doing that, I looked down toward the ocean and said, "We should be going home pretty soon because it's going to get dark."

He said, "Yeah, I know. You just keep picking the food and I'll call you when I'm ready."

So I did that for a while longer. When I stopped again to look for him he wasn't there. I said, "Okay, Grandpa, we're not going to play hide-and-seek because we have to start going down the mountain. If we don't, we're going to get stuck up here."

I kept calling him and he didn't answer. Then I realized he had left me by myself. I had no blankets, no mats to sleep on, nothing. I was angry and scared. I kept saying, "Wait until I get back, Grandpa. I'm going to beat you up, I'm going to kick you, I'm going to punch you." I was trying to be strong, but I was very upset that my grandfather had left me there to survive on my own.

I slept on *hāpu'u* ferns in the lean-to, and the next morning when I got up I heard a loud grunting noise and saw a big pig. I thought she was going to eat me, but I bravely said to her, "Go get your children and bring them here because I'm going to start a Hawaiian class."

She left and, lo and behold, two hours later, I heard squealing and there was the pig, pushing her five babies toward me. I said, "Thank you! Now they can be students in my class." I was thinking I had to do something to keep myself from going crazy; if there was no one else to talk to, I would talk to the little pigs.

During the day, they sat with me, and I taught them the alphabet and the Hawaiian language, and they oinked like they understood what I was saying. At night, they slept in a semicircle outside the opening of the lean-to like they were my bodyguards. For three weeks I lived in the mountains, eating fruits, berries, ti leaf shoots, and whatever else I could find, drinking water I had collected from leaves, and with the pigs for company.

Then one day I felt a hand on my shoulder, and I jumped high in the air. My grandfather caught me. I was so angry when I saw him! I kicked him in the stomach, hit him on the side of his head, and yelled at him.

He hugged me, kept hugging me, and said, "Now we are going home."

I thanked the pigs and said good-bye to them, and my grandfather carried me down the mountain in silence. When we got home, he said, "I took you up there for a reason. That was part of your training. You got the *mana*; you got the power for healing. I'm going to teach you things you need to know, things that are going to help you."

And that's how I started learning about the healing arts.

Nerita Machado
Captain Cook, Island of Hawaiʻi

Although lomilomi *has been practiced by the Hawaiians for centuries, Nerita Machado's mother, "Auntie" Margaret Machado, is credited with bringing it to the forefront of the islands' current health and wellness movement. Every top spa in Hawaiʻi offers* lomilomi *treatments; in fact, many of their therapists were trained either by Auntie Margaret or her protégés. Nerita Machado, a registered nurse, didn't start learning* lomilomi *from her mother until she was forty-two. Today, she is the primary instructor at Hawaiian Lomilomi Massage: A Native Hawaiian Art and Cultural Practice, which was founded by her mother in 1972. The four-week beginners' program consists of weekday workshops from 8:00 a.m. to 5:00 p.m, with a steam bath and* hoʻoponopono *before sunset. Students learn and live together at the Machados' century-old beach house in Keʻei.*

When my mother was sixteen, she fell off a ladder. Because of injuries she received from that accident, she had numbness in her hands and pain in her back and legs. When my sisters and I were small children and didn't weigh much, we massaged her by walking up and down on her back, legs, thighs, buttocks, wherever she told us to go. She would lie facedown in the hallway, we'd put our hands against the wall to support ourselves, and we would walk on her. We didn't massage her with our hands; we walked on her body and pounded her legs until she felt better.

I received my nursing degree from Walla Walla College in Washington State in 1963, then lived and worked in Portland, Oregon, and Glendale, California, for the next twenty-eight years. In 1991, I moved back to the Big Island to help with my mother's *lomilomi* classes.

Only then did I learn that *lomilomi* is committed work; it demands intensive study and dedication. That is what *lomilomi* is about—being kind, patient, understanding, and having unconditional love and acceptance of people for who they are, no matter what.

You've heard the term *hoʻoponopono*, usually defined as a mediation process between parties who are at odds with each other. My mother explained it simply as forgiveness. Before the sun goes down, you need to empty your heart and mind of negative feelings you may have toward yourself, relatives, friends, employers, coworkers, teachers, everyone. If you feel someone has wronged you, you need to ask God to help you forgive that person.

For years my mother's prayer was "Please forgive me if I've sinned against you in thought, word, or deed." That pretty much covers everything. By doing this, she said, you can get into the right spirit for *lomilomi*. This is very important because *lomilomi* is light, gentle, sensitive touch—a connection between heart, hand, and soul. It is a loving touch. Love flows from your heart through your hands to the person you are massaging. In that way, your soul touches their soul.

Hoʻoponopono affects how you touch the person. If you're going through a lot of stress and trauma in your life, you can't concentrate and people will feel it in your massage. You have to have a pure, peaceful, giving heart to do this kind of work. My mother taught that when you give *lomilomi* to people, you should "love their body as if it were your own."

When I teach students, I emphasize that *lomilomi* is not a technique; it's not just physical manipulation. You can learn massage techniques anywhere. Authentic *lomilomi* incorporates both physical and spiritual elements.

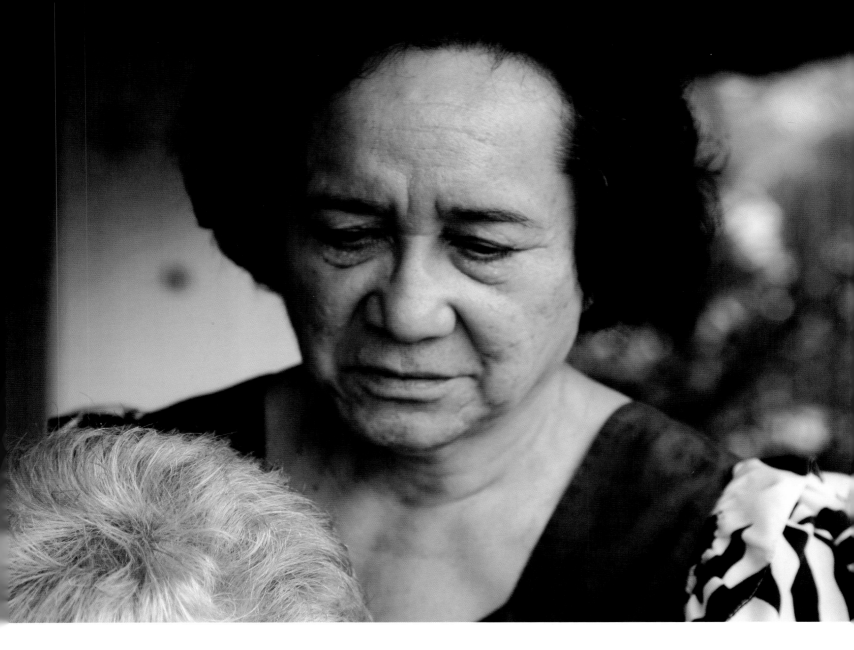

There is no one correct way to do *lomilomi*; in the old days every family had their own way of doing it, although there are some basic principles. You do need a solid background in anatomy and physiology—the nerves, muscles, bones, and joints—otherwise you can hurt people. *Lomilomi* uses a lot of rhythmic, circular movements to get the blood flowing through the body, which is the key to healing.

Often we have students who've gone to other classes and graduated from massage school, but they will say,

"Something is missing in my work." What's missing is the spiritual aspect. They can find this if in their hearts they are receptive to it. In our classes, we ask *Ke Akua* [God] for guidance. We share passages from the Bible from time to time. All students learn the Lord's Prayer in Hawaiian. *Lomilomi* is praying work. I always tell them, "God heals people, God heals the body. We are just the facilitators."

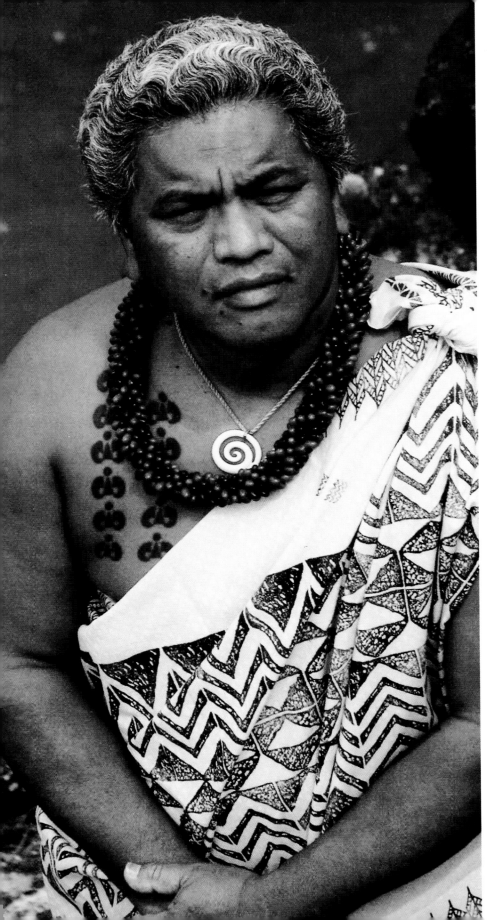

Clifford Nae'ole
Wailuku, Maui

Clifford Nae'ole counts his grandparents—pure Hawaiian on his paternal side, Portuguese and Filipino on his maternal side—among his most influential teachers. His grandfathers introduced him to the wondrous gifts of nature, including plants that could be used to alleviate ailments such as rash, sore throat, and indigestion. Years later, through his hula *studies, he learned the Hawaiian language; genealogy; and ancient rituals, legends, and chants. Nae'ole's connection with the culture has not always been strong. He worked in California for twelve years as a travel agent and hotel manager. Although he was making a good living, he didn't feel fulfilled. Stuck in heavy traffic on Interstate 5 one day in 1989, he realized he'd had enough. He and his family packed up their belongings and came home to Maui for good.*

I learned about medicinal plants in a roundabout way. When I cut down some bushes or mowed down what I thought were weeds, I would get a tongue-lashing from my grandparents. For example, they would say, "Oh, no! That's *pōpolo*! That's one of the most important medicines. You can use it for asthma, cuts, wounds, many things. When you cut it down, you destroy something that can help you."

Those "lessons," however brief, stayed in my mind. From then on, whenever I'd pass a *pōpolo* bush, I would think, *That's* pōpolo, *and it's used as medicine.*

That's how I learned. In those days, anything Hawaiian was subjugated, and my grandparents were chastised for perpetuating the old ways. They never taught us kids per se; I guess they had been humiliated and discouraged when they followed tradition, so it was up to us to watch them and learn on our own.

At the time, my grandparents felt the Hawaiian culture was dying and the way of the future was going to be the Western way. There was no use looking back. They were resigned to that, and wanted us to be able to be on the same footing with our peers and be successful. So although Hawaiian practices were there when I was growing up, they were not ingrained in me. I learned in bits and pieces.

I understand the pain my grandparents must've felt to submerge everything they had been taught. It was that way with other families, too, and, unfortunately, that meant a lot of information about Hawaiian medicine has been lost over the years as the old-timers have passed away. What I did learn from my grandparents made a big impression on me—only I didn't fully realize what I had until years later, when they were all gone.

My renaissance came about relatively recently—in the 1990s when I started learning *hula*. With *hula* comes history, language, and chants, and the doors busted wide open after that. It was only then that I discovered and started understanding that there are so many facets of being a Hawaiian.

Certain things, like burial practices and locations, should be kept *huna* [secret] because they are very sacred. Other things, such as plant medicine, can and should be taught to anyone who's interested in learning. Connecting with nature is an important part of healing. Some *'aumakua* manifest themselves as plants. Our ancestors return as part of nature to help us; we make concoctions from them and take them into our bodies to heal.

In ancient times, after the rains fell, the healers would gather the droplets that had been caught by taro leaves to use for potions because they were pure; they had not touched the earth, which contained the sins of man.

For the same reason, the water of the coconut also was considered pure and used for medicines.

Our *kūpuna* are everywhere in nature to help us. If we pollute the ocean, cut down the trees, we are killing our *kūpuna* and, ultimately, ourselves.

The only way we will survive is to teach the children. In years gone by, you wouldn't see kids playing the *'ukulele*. Now I'm happy to see many of them playing the *'ukulele*. The same thing needs to be done with the healing arts. The old practitioners need to draw children under their wing so they don't mow down the *pōpolo* and other plants that can help us. Teach the young ones what it means to be Hawaiian and inspire them to carry on those ways.

Kapi'ioho'okalani Lyons Naone
Kīpahulu, Maui

Kapi'ioho'okalani Lyons Naone was raised by his grandmother from soon after he was born until he went to O'ahu at age fourteen to attend Kamehameha Schools. He began watching her prepare herbal concoctions when he was six, and although he didn't realize it at the

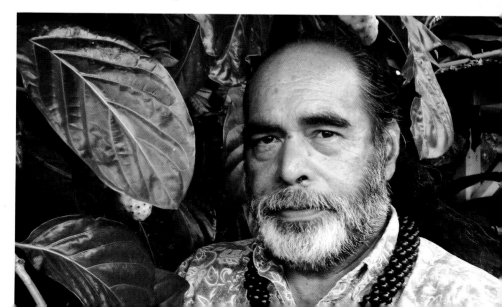

time, that was the beginning of his training. Interestingly, Naone recalls, his grandmother understood the value of blending Christian and traditional Hawaiian practices and philosophies, and he grew up honoring both as well. In addition, respected Hawaiian healers such as Kahu Kawika Ka'alakea, Papa Kalua Kaiahua, Papa Henry Auwae, and Papa Henry Mitchell played influential roles in his life. Naone currently teaches Hawaiian culture and history classes at Maui Community College, and often is asked to give presentations, conduct blessings, and lead workshops throughout Hawai'i, on the mainland, and abroad.

I learned by observing. As a small kid, I didn't really understand everything, but I didn't forget. Then when certain situations came up, I thought, *Oh, I remember; Grandma used to do this and that.*

According to the old Hawaiian way of teaching, knowledge is personally experienced. You look for information yourself, you don't just memorize it.

That's the problem we have nowadays with young healers; they read and that's it. They think doing research is enough. They say, "I've done my research so I'm justified in making these conclusions." Anytime somebody tells me that, I say, "Well, I guess you didn't look then. All you did was research." The Hawaiians say, "'Ike maka—see for yourself."

As far as potential practitioners go, I look for kids who are inquisitive. They don't necessarily ask questions, but they experiment and analyze things. You know kids who eat dirt? Most people would say, "Why are you doing that? What's wrong with you?" but I think that's a good thing; here's a kid who's finding out for himself that dirt tastes bad.

Healing takes into account both the physical and spiritual. People often don't realize that healing comes from within. They say, "I did this chant and that procedure, so I'm taking care of the spiritual part," but, in actuality, they haven't; they've just done "things." Doing things is great, but if they didn't come from within then all you've done is sprinkled water around or waved a feather. You may as well have done the same things with a pom-pom.

I teach people to be more forgiving and tolerant to reduce the stress and anxiety in their lives. Stress and anxiety block the flow of energy in the body, which causes us to be out of balance and alignment, which, in turn, causes illness. To attain and maintain good health, all indigenous peoples recognize the same need to breathe deeply, to relax, to let the energy—the *hā*—flow throughout the body. That centers you, heals you.

When I treat people, I start by focusing on the reason for their anxiety. When their spiritual and emotional problems are addressed, then the physical healing can take place. People may say, "I'm free of pain," but that doesn't mean they're free of illness. Physical symptoms usually aren't the cause of the illness; for a permanent cure, you have to concentrate on the cause.

I don't heal people; they heal themselves with the help of *Akua*. Pleasure is the first form of healing. Getting as much pleasure as you can is healthy. Laugh, have fun, enjoy yourself without abusing your body or putting other people in danger. Soon you'll start feeling "in balance." That's called *pono* in Hawaiian. Most healers say this is the most important ingredient in healing.

How do you find a true healer? A *kahuna* is not going to tell you he's a *kahuna*. He's someone with a vast amount of knowledge and abilities. He's also someone who walks around with a big, empty cup, meaning he's always seeking to have his cup filled with *mana'o* [knowledge]. He knows that no matter how gifted a healer he is, he doesn't know everything. In fact, the more he knows, the bigger and emptier his cup is—the more he realizes he has to learn.

I believe a *kahuna* has paid his dues. He has gone through the rituals of passage of being the servant, being humble and respectful of his elders; then being the student, observing and learning from them; then being the worker, putting his knowledge into practice for the good of other people.

Levon Ohai
Kapa'a, Kaua'i

When Levon Ohai accompanied his "Tutuman" (grandfather), Kaua'i's senior fish and game warden, on field excursions, it was not only a grand adventure, it was a valuable learning experience. His grandfather was responsible for finding lawbreakers—those who caught fish that were too small, who went hunting out of season, and such—and they patrolled wilderness regions throughout the island. On these treks, which often lasted for several hours, his Tutuman would point out various trees and plants to young Ohai, explaining their many uses in ancient times. Thanks to him, Ohai, a seventh-generation herbal healer, says he was well grounded in the basics by the time he was seven. In 2001, he began teaching the only curriculum in the world for traditional Hawaiian herbal healing at the University of Hawai'i at Mānoa.

My Tutuman taught me about herbal medicine because he said I had the personality and temperament of a healer—that is, being slow to anger, slow to judge, well disciplined, and diplomatic. It's not what you say, it's

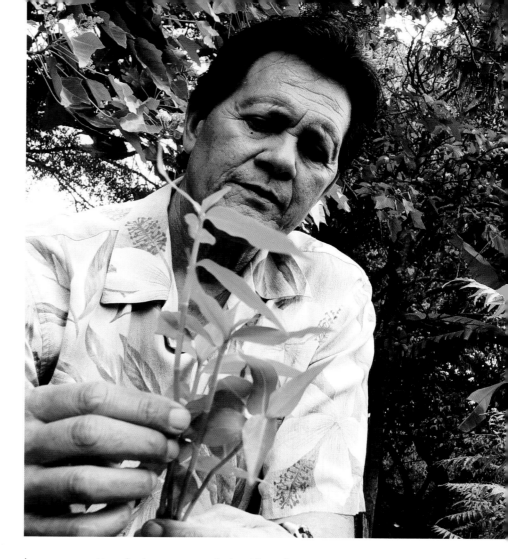

how you say it—whether you can do it without hurting anyone's feelings. Some people will come straight out and say, "You're sloppy, you're lazy, you can't do anything right." But in the old days, the masters never said such things.

You can tell real healers by the way they conduct themselves—the way they say and do things, their knowledge, their lifestyle. They live by what they preach. For example, if they drink and smoke, how can they be warriors carrying the message of healing to people who are sick when they are sick themselves?

Healing is not only about intelligence, it's about intuition—that special sixth sense. So often these days, medical practitioners listen with their ears. In ancient times, they listened with their heart. That's the difference. Today, medicine is completely separate from spirit. It doesn't involve feelings; it's using the brain without the heart, it's a mechanical order of things.

With healing, you not only have to have empirical, factual knowledge, you have to have an inborn trait or spirituality that sharpens your intuition; you'll know by the spirit what is right and what is wrong, and when to do something and when not to do it.

I started going out in the field with Tutuman when I was five. I enjoyed doing that because we'd go to all these beautiful places and I liked seeing different things—the birds, the trees, the 'ōpae [shrimp] in the streams. Tutuman would casually share his wisdom with me, saying, "You see these pōpolo berries? Their juice can be used to clean cuts and wounds," or, "Look at the noni leaves. A tea brewed from them is a good tonic." Although I wasn't really interested in those things at the time, they stuck in my mind because he kept repeating them to me.

Tutuman administered herbs whenever someone in my family got sick. I grew up with herbal medicine. I've only gone to a Western doctor a few times in my life when I've had to in order to play sports, get into college, teach at the university. I've never taken Western drugs, not even aspirin, and I've never had a personal physician. In fact, I've never had any serious illnesses.

Over the years I've come to realize that physical health is closely connected to inner health. The key to healing is not the disease, but why you have the disease. Pressure, stress, and worry change the chemical balance of your body.

Also, because of their hectic lives, people are now eating a lot of unhealthy fast food, whereas when I was growing up, dinner was at six o'clock and the whole family had

better be at the table. Mom spent a lot of time preparing the meal and it was very tasty and nutritious. Everyone talked about what they did that day.

With the breakdown of the family unit has come a breakdown of health. It's an epidemic that has affected every part of America. The good thing is there's a growing interest in and acceptance for natural medicine, which has been around since time immemorial. What we Hawaiian healers are trying to do is to restore it to its proper place.

Marie Place
Manae, Moloka'i

Marie Place's interest in herbal medicine began in 1935, when she was seven years old. She knows that with certainty because that was the year her younger brother John, then five, was thrown off a horse and broke his arm in three places. Place watched her mother prepare a salve of hinahina e kū kahakai *(a beach heliotrope) and* oī *(a kind of verbena) in a container, praying throughout the process. For five straight days, her mother rubbed the concoction on his arm, morning and evening, before wrapping it in cloth. On the sixth day, her mother removed the bandage for the last time. Amazed, Place saw that John's arm had healed perfectly; he could move it without any pain or difficulty, and there was no sign it had ever been broken.*

That really made an impression on me. From then on, I watched my mom closely and wanted to learn her healing practices. I think I knew all of them by the time I was twelve. My mom, who was pure Hawaiian, learned the remedies from her mom who learned them from her mom. That's how knowledge was passed on in those days.

I wanted to write the information on paper, but my mom hit me on the head and said, "No! You never write them

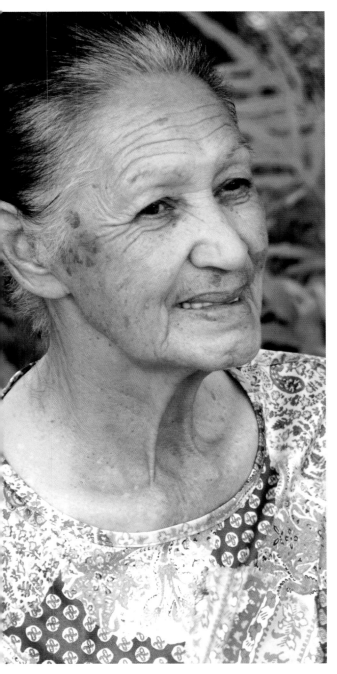

on paper because you're going to put that paper here or there, and you'll wind up losing them. Instead, you keep everything in your head. It will stay there."

So that's why I don't have anything written down. It's all in my head—all the healing plants, where you find them, what they're good for, and how you're supposed to prepare them. I remember it all.

When my brothers and I were children and we got sick, my mom always used plants to treat us—'uhaloa [waltheria] for sore throat, pōpolo [black nightshade] for coughs, laukahi [broad-leafed plantain] for asthma. She showed me plants in our yard—which ones were for medicine and which ones were not. In those days you could find medicinal plants growing everywhere on Moloka'i.

Over the years, they became harder to find, but today they are starting to come back because there's a renewed interest in herbal medicine and people are planting them again. I cannot plant. I tried to plant things, but they wouldn't grow. The kūpuna said if I'm gifted in healing, I wouldn't be able to grow anything. They said I should use my energy to help people, not to plant. Let others do the planting.

In the 1960s, Papa Henry Auwae came to Moloka'i from the Big Island to teach a class. One of the things he taught us was how to prepare coconut milk for healing. He said, "Grate the coconut like you're going to make haupia [pudding]. You squeeze it and strain it, and you put the milk in a pot and cook it on very, very low heat. For two hours you stay there and stir it." I did that and watched how the milk turned clear like water—that really surprised me!

That coconut oil is good for any part of your body that's hurting. When you have stomach problems, you rub it on your stomach. If you have a sore back, you rub it on your back. You only need very little of it.

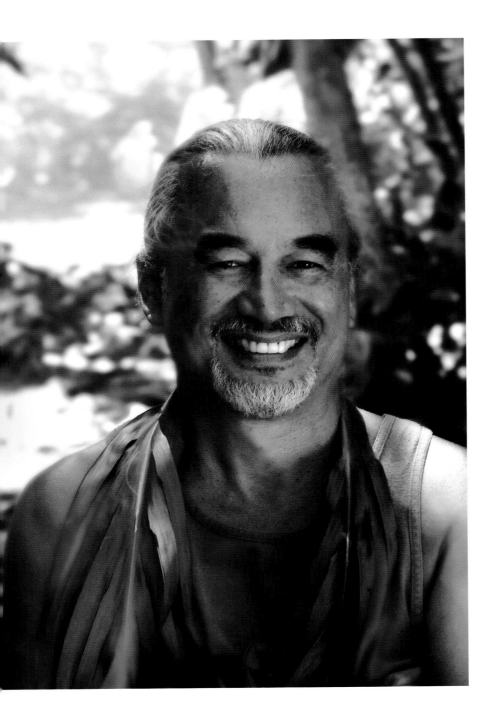

Papa Auwae said it could be stored in the refrigerator. It turns back to the milky color when it's chilled, but if you take it out of the refrigerator the night before you use it, it will be clear in the morning. I still have the same small jar of coconut oil that I made when Papa taught us. I've used it for over forty years and it's still good because I've kept it in the refrigerator.

I always pray when I'm asked to heal, so the treatment that I'm giving people will work. My mom taught me to always pray, to always ask our Heavenly Father to help in the healing process. After all, most of the healing comes from prayer; the plants just help the prayer.

As far as teaching others goes, I don't mind sharing information, but for someone to use that with the intention of making money from it—that's a no-no. Such knowledge should be used to help people, not to make yourself rich. It doesn't matter to me whether you're Hawaiian or Chinese or *haole* (Caucasian), as long as you use what you learn with the right intent, that's fine.

Dane Ka'ohelani Silva
Hilo, Island of Hawai'i

As an elementary-school-age boy, Dane Ka'ohelani Silva often massaged his father, who suffered pain and stiffness from working long hours as a lineman for Hilo Electric Light Company. He doesn't recall who recognized his special gift, but he began training at that time, first with his grandmother, then with his neighbors in Keaukaha, who also were masters of the healing arts. Silva remembers delivering newspapers at age ten to people who would become his mentors. He says there are five basic components of the Hawaiian style of learning: nānā (observe); ho'olohe (listen, obey); pa'a ka waha (literally "shut your mouth" and focus on the things that you are looking at and listening to); nīnau (ask appropri-

ate questions); and hana ka lima (use your hands, do the practical side of the lesson).

I continued to study massage and herbal medicine throughout intermediate and high school, then my training expanded to the martial arts. My uncle explained that the individual who achieved mastery of both the healing and warrior arts was considered to be at the highest level of achievement in the culture.

For two hundred years, the Hawaiian systems of thought and healing were neglected in favor of the Western technology-based philosophy. Traditional cultural practices went deep underground, and only since the 1970s have they again come to light. Many in the Hawaiian community have criticized those, including me, who have revealed some of that traditional knowledge.

But I support the belief of my mentors who said that knowledge about healing and self-protection should be shared in order to help everyone, not only Hawaiians. To prevent selfish abuse of this wisdom, though, I and other Hawaiians follow the tradition of admitting only qualified students to advanced levels of knowledge. Humility is an essential quality for the serious student. A gifted student whose egocentrism causes him to denigrate others in his pursuit of prestige and personal power is recognized as a person who is not qualified for admission to the deeper levels of initiation.

In the context of healing, huna [literally "hidden secret"] is a way to achieve a deeper understanding of the sacred mysteries of life. The five components of learning and mastery are applied in the art of healing to diagnose, treat, and supervise the ongoing care of the patient.

Huna is derived from sacred teachings that had been kept secret for many generations. It existed long before

the kapu [ancient system of laws] was lifted and Christianity began to dominate the life of the Hawaiians.

Today, Western healing is primarily high tech, low touch, and high cost. In ancient times, "technology" didn't exist in machines, transistors, and silicon devices, but in the use and mastery of the mind, body, and spirit. A strong relationship with nature, for example, helped to provide the low-tech, high-touch benefits of exercise, meditation, and medicinal plants. Using their deeper knowledge and higher skills, the kāhuna lā'au lapa'au were able to do many miraculous things. They achieved lōkahi [unity] in their relationships with their people, the environment, and with Akua.

"Technique" is what most students want and are taught—what everybody sees and what they think is most important in healing. As students mature in the arts, however, they begin to understand more of the philosophies of Hawaiian healing. Kuleana: Do the patients accept the primary responsibility for their healing? Pono: Are the patients willing to correct and balance their behavior or lifestyle to overcome diseases of the mind, body, and spirit? Aloha: Is the healer motivated by the higher principles of unconditional caring? Mana: Does the healer possess the level of spirituality that can manipulate the flow of energy that is required by the patient for a successful healing experience?

Although huna is not yet a visible part of the contemporary mainstream of the healing arts, mana is the ingredient that differentiates one healer from another. The more spirituality a practitioner has, the greater his ability to help people heal themselves.

The Hawaiian protocol is to reserve the mana until someone comes and asks for help. People have to ask for help, accept it, believe in it, and take responsibility for their own healing—become an integral part of the healing process.

Knowledge is power. With power comes responsibility. Use it wisely. Live *aloha*.

Ramsay Taum
Honolulu, Oʻahu

Early 1960s. Hawaiʻi had become a state a few years earlier. Although Ramsay Taum's kūpuna *could speak Hawaiian, they didn't whenever he and his siblings were around. Instead, they encouraged him to master English in order to be "successful." By the late 1970s, Taum was interested in reconnecting with his Hawaiian roots. He began with* hula, *learning from renowned* kumu hula *Robert Cazimero and Wayne Chang, who taught cultural principles as well as dance steps. After graduating from Kamehameha Schools and earning a degree in public administration from USC, he learned from esteemed mentors, including Richard Lyman Jr., Pilahi Paki, Donald Kilolani Mitchell, Tommy Solomon, John Dominis Holt III, and Morrnah Simeona, who introduced him to* hoʻoponopono. *Today, Taum guides others through this healing process.*

In 1986, Auntie Morrnah invited me to attend a special *hoʻoponopono* workshop for the National Park Service at Puʻuhonua o Hōnaunau on Hawaiʻi Island. According to her, *hoʻoponopono* is a process of releasing stress by "making things right spiritually"; you might call it spiritual cleansing.

Basically, individuals experiencing *hukihuki* [tension] learn to release unconscious memories that cause and create stress, discomfort, and "dis-ease." *Ponopono* means "neat, arranged, and in order." *Hoʻoponopono* is the process of bringing back proper order, rhythm, balance, and alignment physically, mentally, and emotionally when one is *pono ʻole* [out of balance].

Hoʻoponopono is not something you "do" to others; it is very much a personal, internal thing. Because each person has his or her own blueprint and rhythm, there is no set time for the process or results. Depending on how deep one goes, some people experience results immediately, while others may take longer.

You achieve *hoʻoponopono* by integrating and connecting with your three "inner selves"—your mental, emotional, and spiritual states. Introspection is key. It's about being quiet and mindful. If you were to walk into a *hoʻoponopono* session in progress, the participants might appear to be asleep.

While in that quiet place, you can mentally and spiritually release and remove unconscious memories that trigger negative thoughts and feelings. Upon removing these negative vibrations, mind, body, and spirit become *pono*—integrated. The result of this alignment is being in balance. Where there is balance, there is *pono*. Where there is *pono*, there is no *hukihuki*.

Imagine finding mold on your ceiling. The cause is a leaky pipe hidden in the walls. Even though you replace the ceiling tiles, the mold returns within a short time. Why? Because rather than fixing the problem, the leak, you only repaired the surface symptom, the mold.

So it is with *hoʻoponopono*. To cleanse one's mind and spirit and let go of the *hukihuki*, you have to reach beyond the surface tension.

To get to the "leak," the source of your tension, you have to *ʻōʻō* [dig] deep into *pō* [dark places] to remove the source of stress. *Hoʻo* refers to the act of combining.

One of the results of *ho'oponopono* is the integration of the three states of your inner self—mental, spiritual, and emotional, or what Auntie Morrnah calls "inner family"—to achieve *pono*. The steps in the process are embedded in the word itself!

The mold on the ceiling didn't appear overnight; the leak, the cause of the mold, went undetected for a long time. Like the leak, *hukihuki* between you and others doesn't just suddenly appear, but often has a history that has been ignored or gone undetected.

It's akin to an onion, consisting of many layers. *Ho'oponopono* helps to peel away those layers, one by one. Each time you remove a layer, another one is revealed, but now you have the ability to deal with that issue and those that might accompany it.

Another important element of *ho'oponopono* is forgiveness. *Aloha* has to be given as much as it is received. There's a reciprocity agreement between participants, as well as with the practitioner.

For example, would you feed your child after working in the dirt without washing your hands first? Similarly, a surgeon is expected to sterilize his hands and arms before operating. *Ho'oponopono* is like doing a spiritual scrub before surgery. If the practitioner doesn't do this, his negative thoughts, emotions, and assumptions could be passed on to others, thus adding to the *hukihuki* rather than reducing it.

Just as you shower to cleanse your body every day, so should *ho'oponopono* be a daily practice to cleanse your mind and spirit.

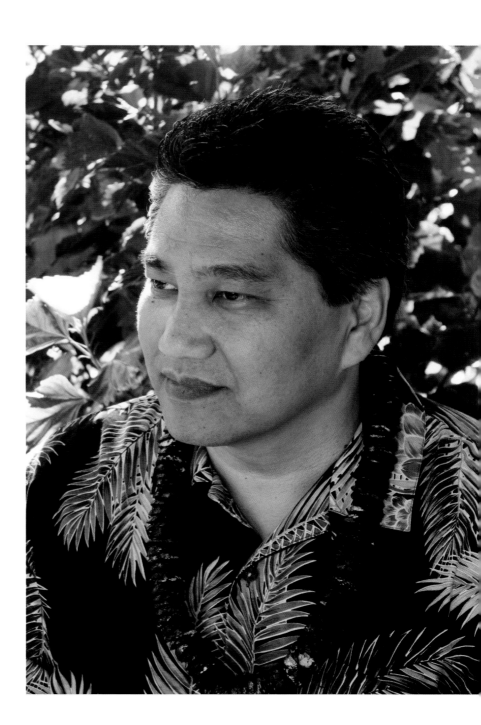

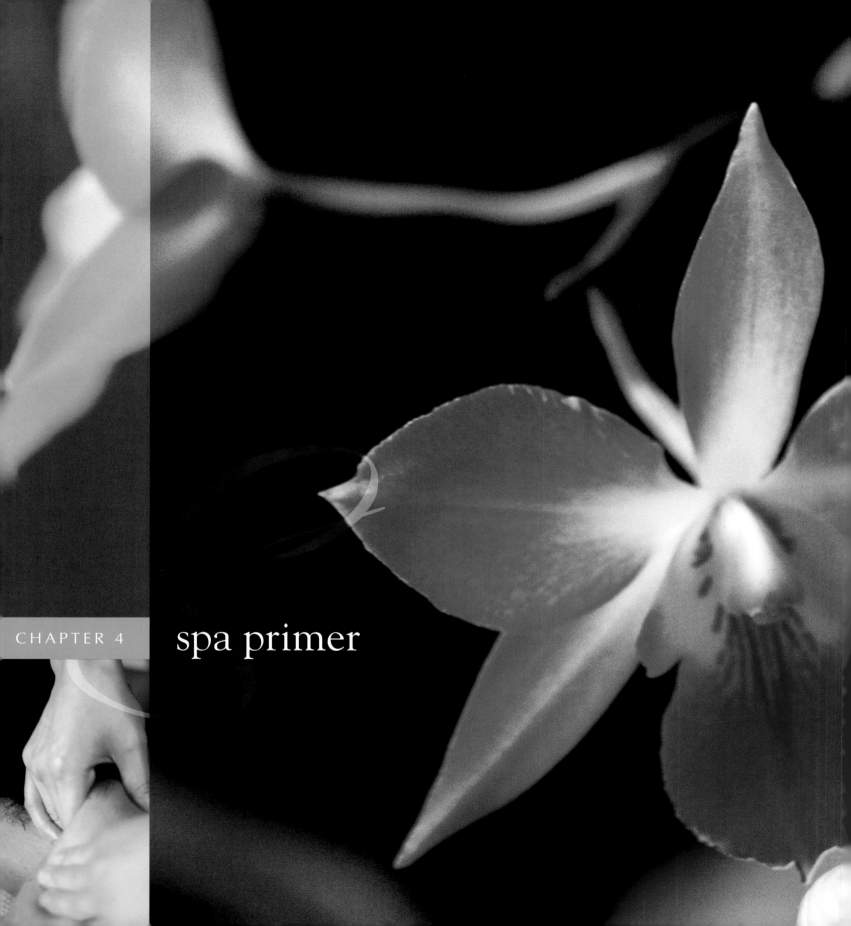

spa primer

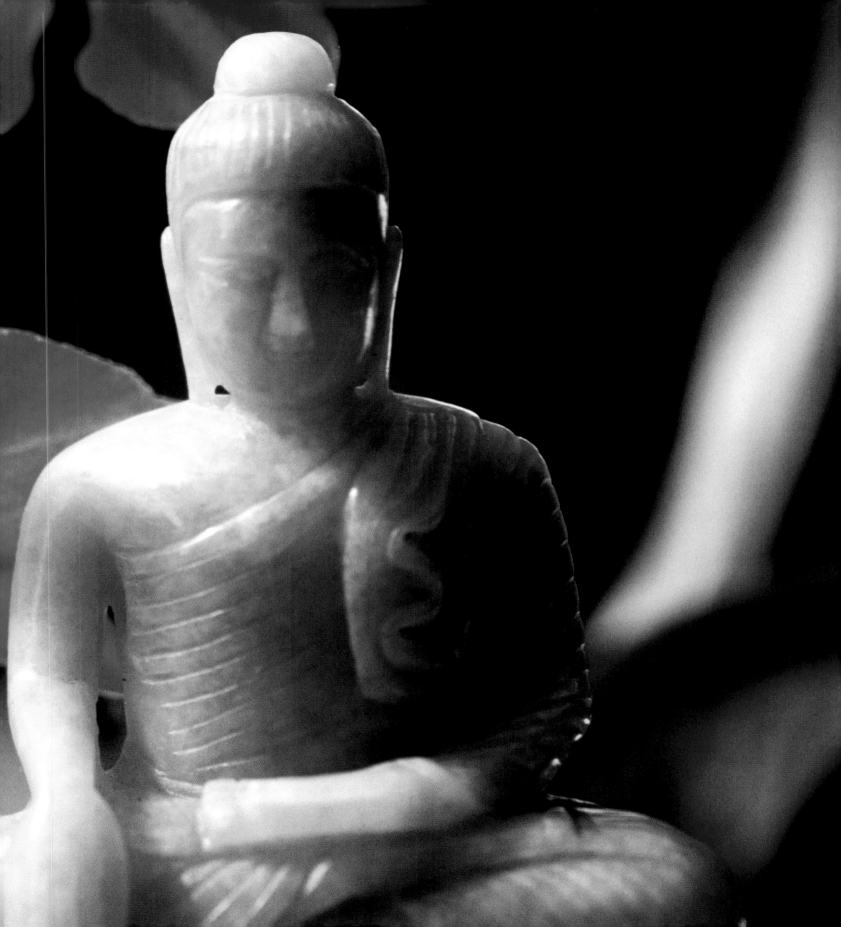

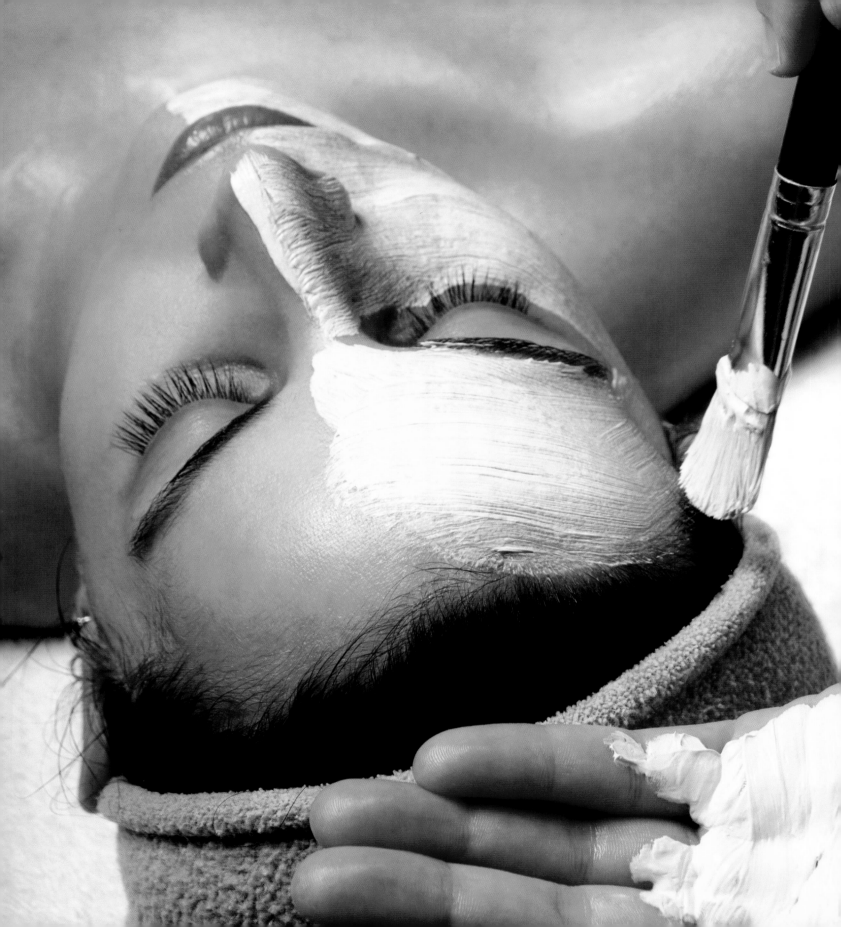

c h a p t e r   4

To the uninitiated, the spa exudes a definite mystique. The fact that people would willingly pay to have strangers smear mud on their faces; rub coarse salt on their skin; and press, stretch, and knead their bodies while they're completely unclothed surely must seem strange. It's no wonder, then, that there are a lot of misconceptions about spas. Among them:

Spas are for the wealthy. While it's true a visit to a top resort spa in Hawai'i will probably cost at least a hundred dollars, you can treat yourself at a neighborhood day spa for much less.

Spas are for women. Currently, about 30 percent of spa customers are men and the number is rising. A few Hawai'i spas even offer treatments that are "just for men."

PRECEDING SPREAD: Fresh flowers and fabulous figurines adorn many of Hawai'i's spas.

LEFT: Skilled estheticians rejuvenate your entire body, from head to toe.

Spas are for old people. A recent study conducted by the International Spa Association (ISPA) reported that nearly four million spa-goers in the U.S. are teenagers. Several Hawai'i spas have created special menus for young children and teens.

Spa visits are an indulgence. According to the ISPA survey, consumers visit a spa for reasons other than mere pleasure, the top three being to relieve stress (47 percent), soothe sore joints and muscles (38 percent), and to feel better about themselves (31 percent).

Spa visits are irregular and infrequent. Not so, says the ISPA research. Seventy-one percent of U.S. spa-goers have been going to spas for at least three years. Moreover, the responses indicated that once people have tried a spa, they are very likely to return.

BELOW: A spa visit can help you feel fresh and beautiful, like a flower in full bloom.

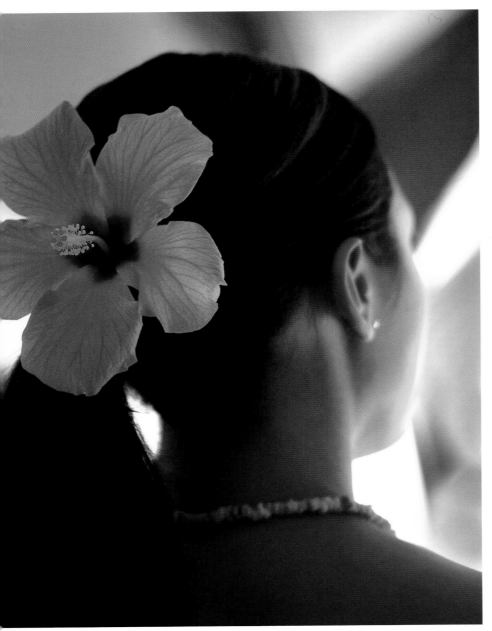

Read on for more interesting tidbits about the spa.

HISTORY OF THE SPA

More than fifteen hundred years ago, battle-weary soldiers of the Roman Empire searched for mineral springs to cleanse their wounds and soothe their aches and pains. Bathing in the warm, tranquil waters lifted their spirits and provided them with a much-needed respite from the horrors of war.

Scholars theorize *spa* is the acronym for the soldiers' descriptions of their restorative time in these springs—*Sanitas Per Aquas*, which translated from Latin means "health through waters"; *Sanare Per Aquam*, "to heal through water"; and *Salut Per Aqua*, "relaxation through water." The word also could be a derivative of *espa*, meaning "fountain," or *spargere*, "to bubble up, sprinkle, or moisten."

During the height of the Roman Empire, around the second century AD, a town in a beautiful wooded area near Liège in eastern Belgium won renown for the healing powers of its mineral springs. It was dubbed Spa, and by the Middle Ages (roughly AD 500 to 1500), patrons by the droves—including kings, aristocrats, statesmen, and poets—were flocking there to experience its miraculous springs.

Throughout the eighteenth and nineteenth centuries, the elite in Europe frequented Spa and other scenic spots blessed with thermal springs. They came to "take the waters"—drink water from the springs; use nutrient-rich mud gathered from the sites for skin treatments; and soak away stress, fatigue, and depression in baths drawn from the warm pools.

The idea for the spa as we now know it can be traced to Germany, where doctors prescribed stays at a *kurot* (place of cure) for patients. These "spa villages" usually were nestled in picturesque alpine or seaside locales, where the temperature, quality of air, and exposure to the sun played key roles in the healing process. Sojourns lasted two to four weeks, during which a doctor oversaw a *kur* (cure) system of natural therapies such as hydrotherapy, massage, herbal and peat hot packs, oxygen and inhalation therapies, and more.

European immigrants brought the *kur* concept to the United States at the turn of the twentieth century. Today, spas no longer are regarded as exclusive haunts for the privileged class, but as mainstream wellness centers that embrace a holistic philosophy—that is, treatment of the whole body (physical, mental, emotional, and spiritual) rather than a few of its ailing parts. Proponents of holistic medicine believe that optimum health is obtained when one's entire being is in harmony.

Thus, the aim of spas is to help renew and invigorate clients through positive lifestyle changes, and, accordingly, menus have expanded to include much more than water-based therapies (see chapter 5: Rest, Relax, Rejuvenate). "Spa" is now synonymous with health, fitness, beauty, tranquility, and renewal.

In fact, spa vacations are growing in popularity. While these escapes tout lovely settings, wonderful amenities, and ample time for leisure, the daily regimen can be quite strict. Guests sometimes stay for several weeks at a time to accomplish predetermined goals such as losing weight, getting in shape, alleviating chronic conditions, dropping bad habits, or learning about nutrition and exercise.

The spa's team of professionals—including medical and naturopathic doctors, chiropractors, nutritionists, estheticians, cosmetologists, psychologists, massage therapists, personal trainers, and first-class chefs—is committed to helping guests achieve long-term physical, mental, spiritual, and emotional equilibrium. They create a customized, integrated course of action; give instruction and encouragement; monitor progress; complete regular assessments; and suggest a maintenance plan that patrons can follow when they return home.

In keeping with their holistic approach to health, some spas offer tennis, racquetball, and volleyball courts; swimming pools; fitness centers; beauty salons; dance studios; and yoga, *tai chi*, Pilates, spinning (stationary indoor cycling), meditation, nutrition, and stress management classes. For many people, spa visits no longer are a luxury; they're essential elements of their overall health plans, providing comprehensive tune-ups that relax, revitalize, boost energy, and promote inner peace.

The Hawaiian spa is unlike any other, anywhere. Treatments and facilities recall ancient cultural traditions, mirror the diversity of the Aloha State's cosmopolitan population, and showcase the tropical beauty of the islands. You can enjoy aqua bodywork in the ocean and massage in a thatched *hale* (hut) set in a vibrant garden. You can indulge in scrubs made of Kona coffee, sea salt, turbinado sugar, or *'alaea* (red clay); and facials and wraps using ti leaves, volcanic ash, or medicinal plants such as *noni* (Indian mulberry), *'ōlena* (turmeric), and *'awapuhi* (wild ginger). Services run the gamut, from Japanese *shiatsu*, Swiss shower, Swedish massage, and Indian *shirodhara* to Chinese acupuncture, Finnish sauna, Thai massage, and Hawaiian *lomilomi*.

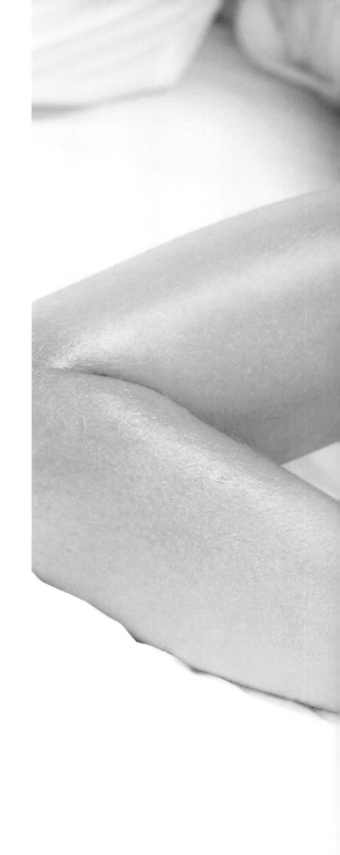

RIGHT: Spa treatments, including massage, help you escape the cares of everyday life for a few blissful hours.

However you choose to spend your time at a spa, you'll find it is a precious gift—an opportunity for you to slow your pace, reexamine your priorities, regenerate your entire being, and rediscover the wonder of you.

SELECTING A SPA

People visit spas for many reasons. Some may just need an hour-long massage or facial to escape the demands of everyday living. Others may sign up for programs that last a week or longer to gain more than momentary relaxation.

To find the facility that best suits your needs, first outline your goals. Do you want to find relief for a nagging physical problem? Are you looking for ways to cope with the pressures of your job and home responsibilities? Is support what you seek as you face a major challenge in your life such as a divorce, serious illness, or death of a loved one? Would you like to lose weight, quit smoking, improve your diet, develop athletic skills, start a regular exercise routine, and adopt other good health habits? Or do you just want to pamper yourself?

Once you've identified what you'd like to accomplish, determine how much time and money you can afford. Also decide on a geographic location; do you prefer a spa by the ocean or the mountains? Is a destination in the desert or the country more appealing? Or, for the sake of convenience, would you rather plan a getaway in your hometown?

There are several other important things to consider before you make a decision, among them the type of program (individualized or group?); accommodations (cabin, cottage, yurt, dormitory, lodge, or swank hotel?); length of stay (flexible or set dates?); schedule (go with the flow or structured?); meals (cafeteria-style or table

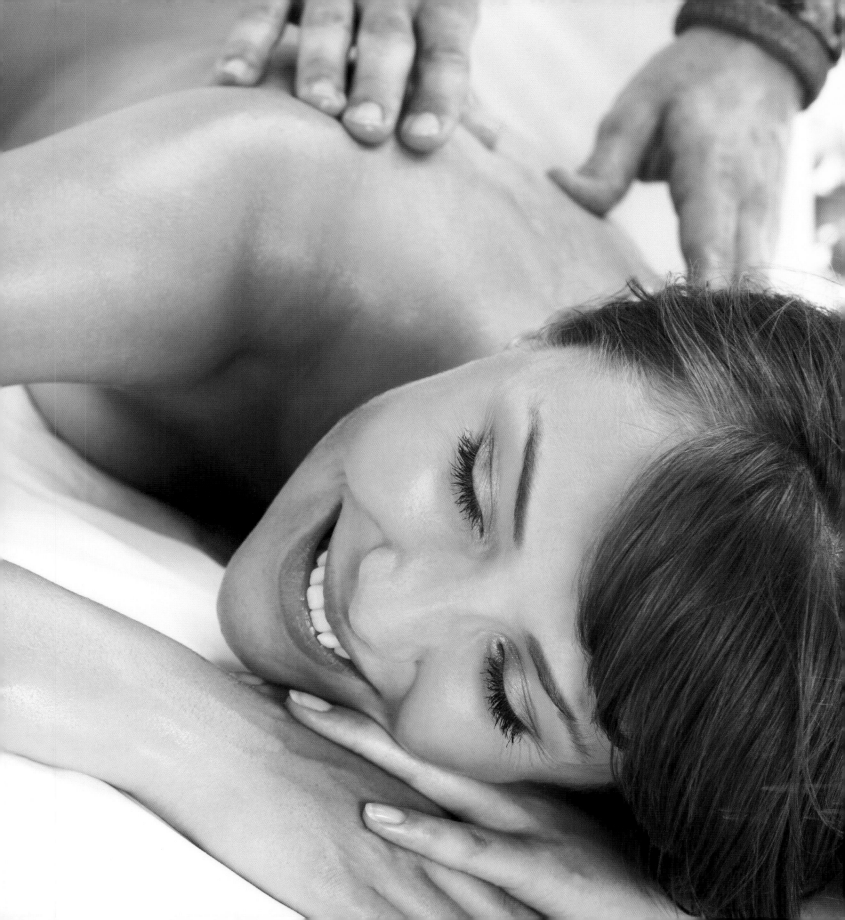

service?); and optional activities (movies, games, parties, sightseeing, shopping?). Information is readily available, so do your homework. Review material in libraries and bookstores. Get recommendations from friends, family members, and coworkers. Conduct research on the Internet. Request brochures from the spas that most interest you, then choose one within your budget that offers the services, setting, activities, and accommodations that you seek.

Founded in 1991 and headquartered in Lexington, Kentucky, the International Spa Association is recognized as the professional organization and voice of the spa industry. It represents more than three thousand health and wellness facilities and providers in seventy-five countries. Members include physicians, nutritionists, massage therapists, product suppliers, and the seven primary types of spas defined on its Web site (www.experienceispa.com) as follows:

Club spa: A facility whose primary purpose is fitness, and which offers a variety of professionally administered spa services on a day-use basis.

Cruise ship spa: A spa aboard a cruise ship providing professionally administered spa services, fitness and wellness components, and spa cuisine.

Day spa: A spa offering a variety of professionally administered spa services to clients on a day-use basis.

Destination spa: A spa with the primary purpose of guiding individual spa-goers to develop healthy habits. Historically a seven-day stay, this lifestyle transformation can be accomplished by providing a comprehensive program that includes spa services, physical fitness activities, wellness education, healthful cuisine, and special interest programming.

Medical spa: A facility that operates under the full-time, on-site supervision of a licensed health-care professional. The professional's primary purpose is to provide comprehensive medical and wellness care in an environment that integrates spa services with traditional, complementary, and/or alternative therapies and treatments. The facility operates within the scope of practice of its staff, which can include both aesthetic/cosmetic and prevention/wellness procedures and services.

Mineral springs spa: A spa offering an on-site source of natural mineral, thermal, or ocean water used in hydrotherapy treatments.

Resort/Hotel spa: A spa owned by and located within a resort or hotel providing professionally administered spa services, fitness and wellness components, and spa cuisine. In addition to the leisure guest, this is a great place for business travelers who wish to take advantage of the spa experience while away from home.

SPA ETIQUETTE

If you haven't been to a spa before, these twelve tips can ensure you have an enjoyable experience.

• Request a menu of the spa's services ahead of time so you can review prices and ask questions about anything that isn't clear. When you make your appointment, you'll need to specify what treatment you'd like so the proper therapist and allotment of time can be reserved for you. This also would be when you should make special requests—such as your preference of a male or female therapist, an indoor or outdoor venue, or a specific oil or lotion fragrance.

• Realize that a spa is a place of peace and quiet designed to remove you from distractions. Don't eat a

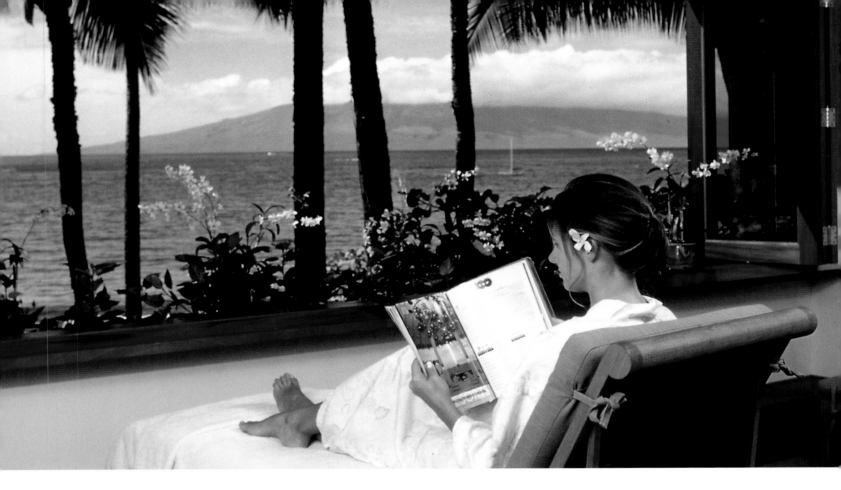

heavy meal before your treatment, leave your laptop and young children at home, turn off your cell phone and pager, and avoid loud conversation when you're there. It's also a good idea not to wear jewelry, as it will have to be removed for your treatment anyway.

• Arrive at least thirty minutes in advance so you have enough time to check in, go on a short tour of the facilities, put your personal belongings in a locker (bring as little as possible), and change. The spa should provide a robe and slippers for you to use while you're there.

• You'll get the most out of full-body treatments if you are nude. Don't fret; your therapist will drape areas that aren't being worked on with a sheet or blanket. If that knowledge doesn't lessen your anxiety, then undress to your level of comfort.

• You may be asked to answer questions about your health, prior injuries, and problem spots. Be honest and as detailed as possible. That's the only way your therapist will be able to determine the best techniques and products to use.

• Shower before your treatment; it starts the decompression process and removes any lotion, sunscreen, perfume, or hair spray so your body can soak up all the beneficial ingredients of your treatment. If you like, slip into the sauna, steam room, hot tub, or whirlpool before heading to the lounge to wait for your therapist. Most spas furnish their lounges with comfortable chairs and sofas, magazines, fresh fruits, chilled water, hot tea, and soothing background music.

• Clear your mind for the treatment. You can worry about deadlines, errands, and other concerns later. Breathing deeply and visualizing things that are dear to you—a special event, place, person, or even pet—also will help you relax.

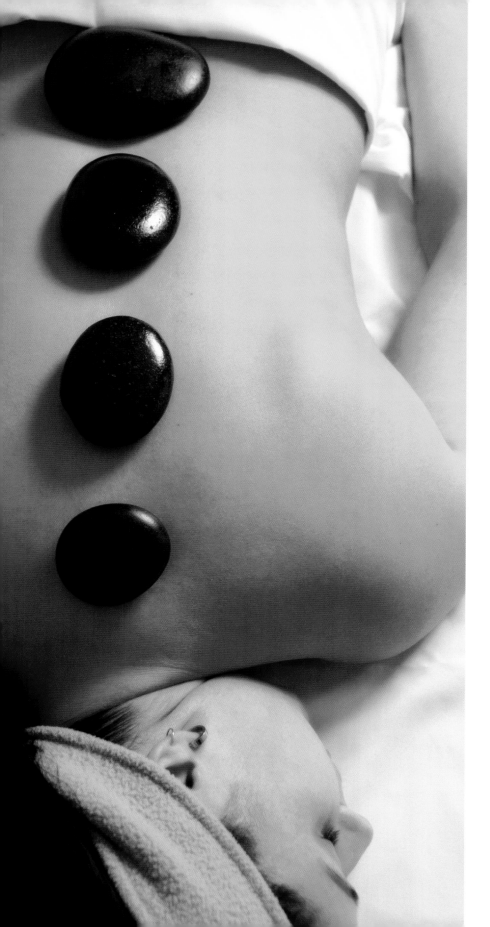

• Some people like to chitchat during their treatments; others don't. Your therapist will take the cue from you—or, even better, you can state your preference up front.

• Provide your therapist with feedback on the lighting and temperature of the room, type and volume of the music, intensity of the pressure, parts of your body that need special attention, and what techniques you do and don't like. Don't be shy about asking questions or discussing your apprehensions. Open communication with your therapist is important.

• You'll know your treatment has ended when your therapist says something like "Please take a few minutes before getting up." You usually can rest where you are for about five minutes before the room needs to be prepared for the next client. Don't pop up too fast or you may feel woozy. If you need more relaxation time, you're welcome to return to the lounge.

• A gratuity of 15 to 20 percent for good service is standard. If you're using a gift certificate, ask if the tip was included. If not, you can give your therapist a cash tip or leave one for him or her at the reception desk, where envelopes usually are available.

• Be sure to drink lots of water throughout the day after your treatment; this will flush out toxins that have been released in your system. Also, don't plan a hectic schedule, which will counteract all the benefits you've received. Instead, engage in quiet pursuits at home such as reading, gardening, writing in your journal, or watching a movie.

YOUR HOME SPA

Can't get away to a spa? Then bring the spa to you! Contrary to what you might think, it's not difficult to create

BELOW: Use candles, aromatherapy, and plush towels to create a spa experience at home.

the nurturing ambience of a spa in your home. Here are a few suggestions.

• Convert a quiet spot, away from highly trafficked areas, into your "spa." It could be a patio; deck; balcony; storage room; large closet; or a corner of your den, bedroom, or living room. Furnish it with a comfortable love seat or chair, a footrest, and a small table.

• If you have an entire room to work with, paint it! Good choices are blue, which reflects peace and stability; green, which soothes and calms; yellow, which is cheerful and uplifting; or earth tones such as ocher, russet, and sage, which create a warm, intimate ambience.

• Fill the area with things you love, including artwork, photos, candles, incense, pillows, and fresh flowers and plants. Have a portable CD player on hand so you can play your favorite relaxation music, whether it be nature sounds, classical music, slack key guitar, or instrumentals. If the room has windows, hang little bells or wind chimes that will tinkle as the breezes blow.

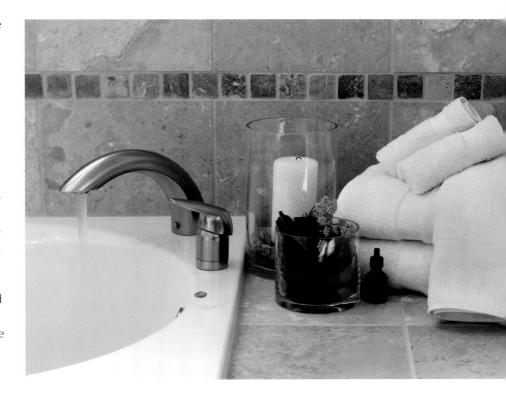

BELOW: Use candles, aromatherapy, and plush towels to create a spa experience at home.

• To enjoy the benefits of aromatherapy, burn incense or place sachets around your haven. You either can buy these perfumed pouches or make your own by filling little organza bags with potpourri, rose petals, or sprigs of lavender. When the fragrance fades, refresh it with a drop of essential oil or a light spray of perfume. You also can purchase diffusers, which release tiny amounts of essential oils in the air.

• The sight and sound of water are very soothing. If space permits, set up an aquarium, fountain, pond, birdbath, or other water feature in your home or yard. It doesn't have to be grand or expensive; in fact, books, Internet articles, and home improvement stores can show you how to do it yourself.

• Invest in tools, supplies, and accessories. A starter list should include loofah sponges and mitts; natural bristle brushes; wooden massage rollers; herbal eye pillows; inflatable neck pillows; pumice stones; nail files; stainless steel, plastic, or ceramic trays; a shower cap; disposable rubber gloves; terry cloth face and hand towels; standard-size and oversize bath towels; several cotton sheets; blankets; house slippers; a comfortable robe; a shower curtain or plastic sheets; fresh flowers; candles; soft music; and your choice of quality beauty products such as soaps, shampoos, conditioners, bath salts, essential oils, lotions, toners, and cleansers.

• Treatments don't have to be elaborate to be effective; for instance, settling in a comfy chair with a good

RIGHT: Your feet deserve pampering, too! Reflexology is based on the belief that pressure points on the feet correspond to major organs.

book, relaxing background music, and a freshly brewed cup of tea can work wonders. Peruse the easy recipes in chapter 8: Beauty from Head to Toe, which call for ingredients you regularly stock in your kitchen. Or try the following simple therapies.

Refreshing Hand Soak
Add a few drops of lemon or lime juice to a basin of warm water. Soak your hands in it for five to ten minutes.

Cool Cucumber Compress
Cut a chilled cucumber into round slices and put one on each closed eyelid to reduce pain and puffiness.

Easy Foot Massage
Place about two dozen marbles or small smooth rocks in a basin of warm water. Roll your feet over them to ease aching muscles.

Milk Mask
Boil two cups of whole milk, then set it aside to cool. A "skin" will form on top of the milk; skim it off and apply it to your face. After it dries, gently scrub it off with a loofah sponge or terry cloth towel.

Red Wine and Honey Relaxer
Fill your bathtub with warm water. Add one cup of honey and four cups of red wine (a cheap one will work fine). Soak in it for twenty minutes.

Fruity Facial
Mash equal parts watermelon, cantaloupe, and honeydew, and apply the mixture to your face. Let it sit for twelve to fifteen minutes, then rinse with warm water and pat dry.

Heavenly Hair Treatment
Dampen your hair and apply conditioner as directed on the bottle. Warm a damp towel in the microwave. Wrap your head in the towel for at least fifteen minutes, allowing the conditioner to be thoroughly absorbed. Remove the towel and wash your hair as you normally do.

Blissful Bath
Remove dead skin cells with a dry brush exfoliation. Draw a warm scented bubble bath or add a few drops of essential oil to a tub filled with warm water. Soak in it for twenty minutes (the experience is even better if you have a whirlpool bath). After drying off with a towel, generously apply a moisturizing body lotion.

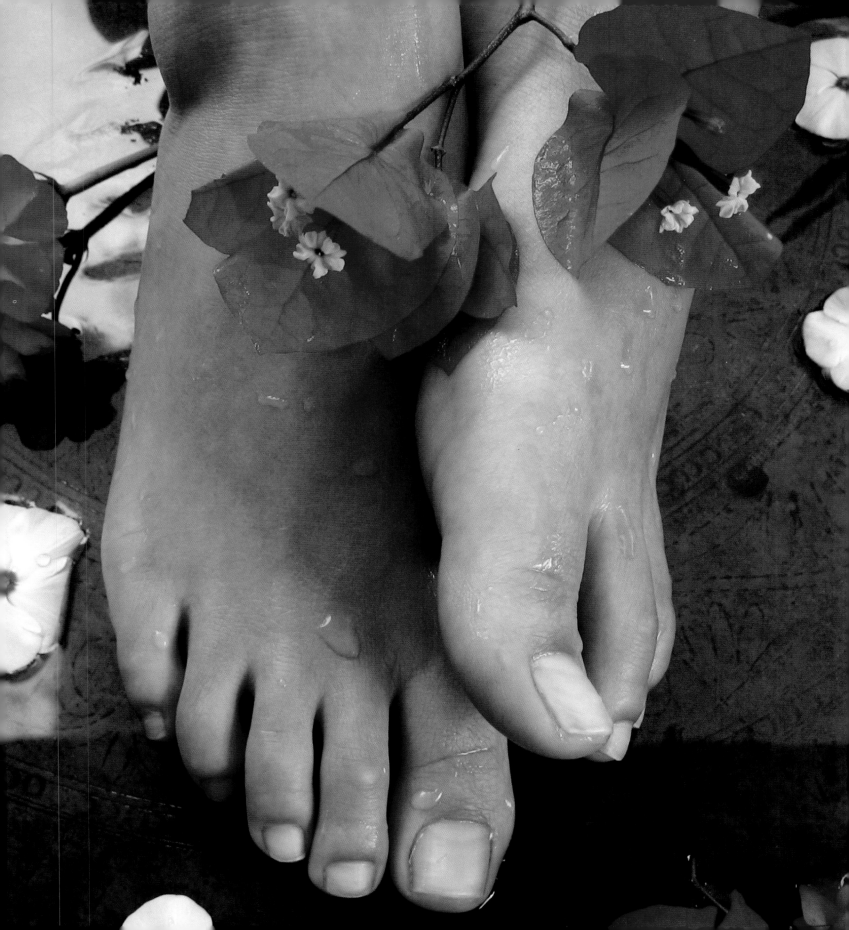

rest, relax, rejuvenate

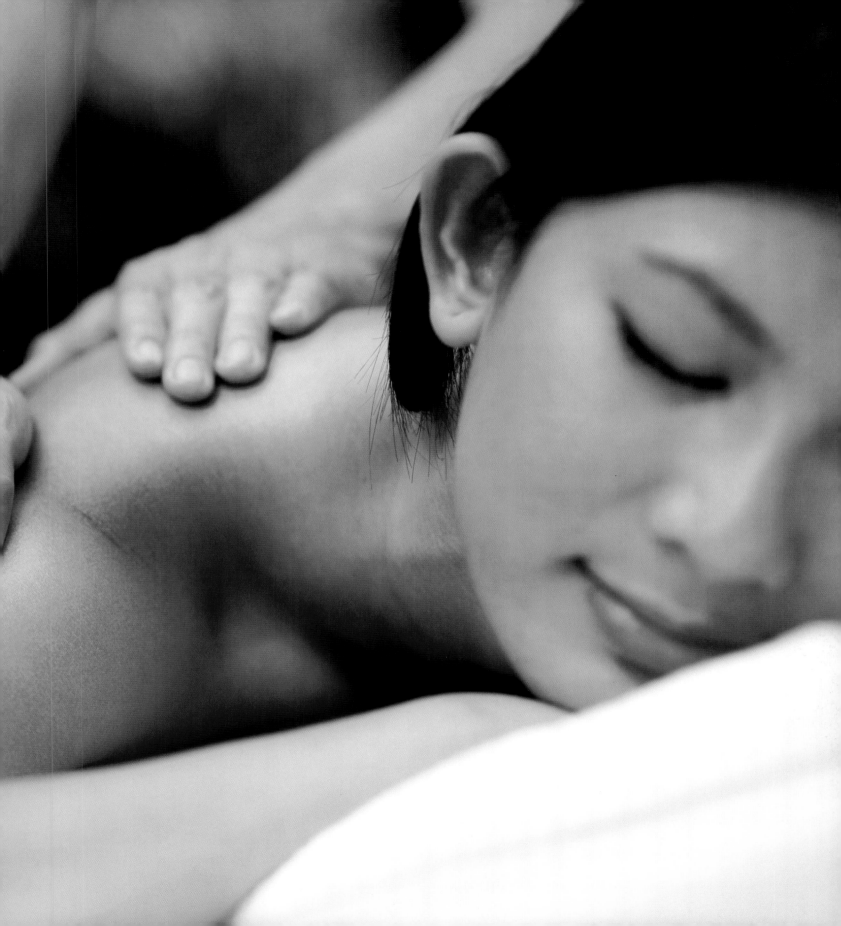

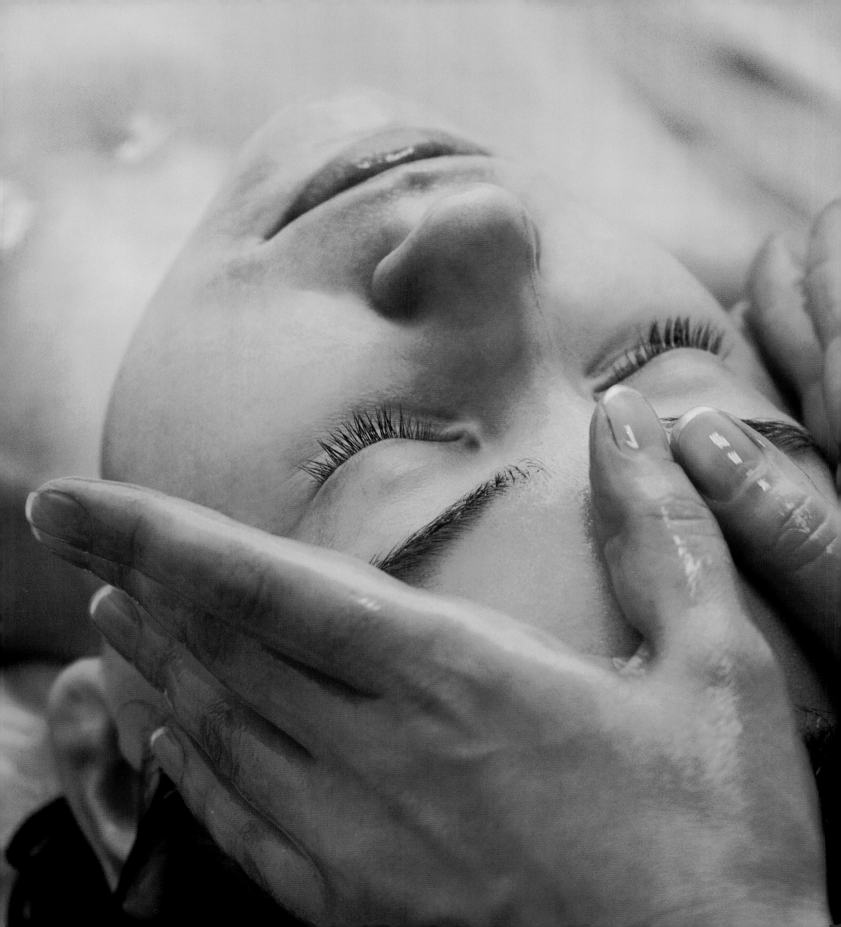

chapter 5

Spas offer many different kinds of treatments to renew body, mind, and spirit. They are classified in these general categories, based on the primary ingredient or technique used:

Aroma: Essential oils
Balneo: Baths
Hydro: Water
Masso/Presso: Manipulation of pressure points
Physio: Any physical or mechanical treatment, including masso/presso
Phyto: Plants
Radon: Inert gas
Thalasso: Seawater and marine by-products
Thermal: Heat, both wet and dry

At a spa, we can shut out everything that's causing us pain, stress, and worry, and focus on ourselves. Healing, after all, starts from within. We all possess the power to aid the healing process; we just may need help channeling it.

PRECEDING SPREAD: Among other things, massage has been shown to alleviate stress, improve circulation, and reduce muscle and joint stiffness.

LEFT: Touch can calm, reassure, uplift, and heal. Massage is the most popular spa treatment in the United States.

Spa treatments relax, revitalize, beautify, and detoxify. They're blissful interludes that put us on the path to optimum health. Even an hour in a spa can make a big difference in your life. Take the time, spend the money. You're worth it.

HEALING WITH TOUCH: MASSAGE

A hug, a kiss, a gentle hand on the shoulder—touch is at once the simplest and most intimate form of communication. Touch calms, reassures, and uplifts. It reminds us we're not alone and says, "I care," "I understand," "I'm here for you," "I believe in you"—and everything that words often can't.

To survive, we humans need to touch and be touched as surely as we need food, water, and sleep. In the womb, touch is the first of our five senses to develop. As soon as we're born, we learn about our new world primarily through tactile experience, and thrive on loving contact with our parents.

Touch is an instinctive response to pain and discomfort. When you have a cramp, sprain, bruise, or other such physical ailment, the natural tendency is to obtain relief by pressing and rubbing it. When people you care about are sad, frightened, or worried, you bolster them with a hug or caress. In fact, touch is one of the oldest known healing modalities.

Massage, the most familiar form of touch therapy, employs the hands and/or instruments to manipulate the soft tissues of the body. As early as 3000 BC, Chinese healers were practicing *amma*, which evolved into the technique we now call acupressure. The *Huang Ti Nei Ching* (Yellow Emperor's Classic of Internal Medicine), a book from that period, recommended *amma* as an effective means of treating disease and maintaining optimum health.

From China, massage spread to India, where the first writings about it, the *Ayur-Veda* (Art of Life), appeared around 1800 BC. This sacred Hindu book introduced a holistic system of healing known today as Ayurveda, including simple massage treatments using fragrant herbs and spices.

Massage went from India to Greece around 1000 BC. Homer, the celebrated Greek poet who wrote the epics *Iliad* and *Odyssey* around 720 BC and 700 BC, respectively, noted massage was part of the therapeutic regimen for warriors who complained of fatigue and muscle pain.

In the fifth century BC, Hippocrates observed, "The physician must be experienced in many things, but assuredly in rubbing . . . for rubbing can bind a joint that is too loose, and loosen a joint that is too rigid." Julius Caesar (100 to 44 BC), Rome's great general and statesman, supposedly was "pinched" every day to alleviate neuralgia, headaches, and epileptic seizures.

Massage currently is the most popular spa treatment in the United States. Licensed massage therapists who are well versed in human anatomy use their hands, forearms, elbows, and even their feet to press, tap, knead, rock, pull, vibrate, and stroke their clients, providing numerous physiological and psychological benefits. Among these are:

- Relaxes the body
- Reduces muscle and joint stiffness, aches, and spasms
- Alleviates headaches, stress, anxiety, and insomnia
- Improves circulation, flexibility, range of motion, and organ function
- Eases chronic pain and swelling
- Calms the nervous system
- Lowers blood pressure and heart rate
- Tones the skin
- Eliminates toxins
- Increases metabolism and concentration
- Releases endorphins, the body's natural painkillers
- Strengthens the immune system
- Relieves depression, grief, and anxiety
- Renews energy and diminishes mental fatigue
- Fosters peace of mind, well-being, relaxation, and contentment

It takes years of education and practice for a professional therapist to locate problem areas, learn all the different massage techniques (there reportedly are dozens of them), determine which ones are appropriate for which conditions, and execute the right amount of pressure. Even so, an untrained person can provide a relaxing, if not curative, massage. On the market are many books that explain and illustrate the basic techniques. To prepare for an informal massage at home, reserve a

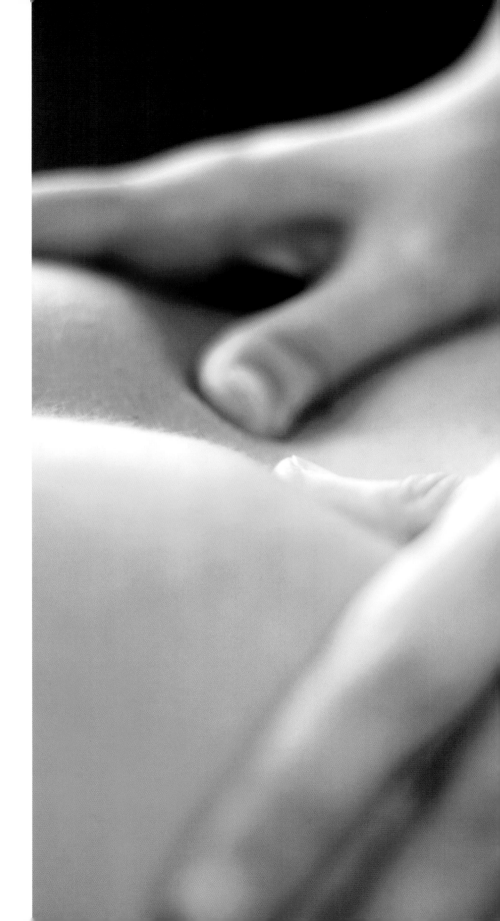

time when you don't have any commitments. You'll receive the most benefits from the session if you're nude; if you must wear clothes, they should be loose, light, and made of cotton, a fabric that breathes.

Choose a quiet spot that's free from drafts and distractions such as kids playing, ringing phones, a blaring TV or radio, and noisy washing machines and dryers. Lighting should be soft and subdued; candlelight or indirect lighting from a floor or table lamp is ideal. Turn on mellow music. To add fragrance, burn incense, set out sachets or a floral bouquet, or add a few drops of essential oil to the melted wax at the top of a flickering candle.

A firm, padded surface such as a futon or mattress is best (a couch is not desirable because it doesn't provide enough support for your body). Elevate the surface so the person who's giving you the massage won't be bending over too much, and make sure there's at least two feet around it so he/she can move about easily. When lying on your stomach, place a rolled-up towel under your ankles to remove pressure from your knees. When you're on your back, you'll feel more comfortable with a small, flat cushion under your head, a pillow under your lower back, and a rolled-up pillow under your knees.

Warmth is essential for massage work; the temperature in the room should be between seventy and seventy-five degrees. If your skin is cold, it will not be supple or absorb lubricants such as cream, lotion, or oil very well. Also, your body temperature will drop during the massage, and when muscles get cold they contract, which will counteract any good you might gain from the treatment. Areas of your body that aren't being massaged should be kept covered with towels or blankets.

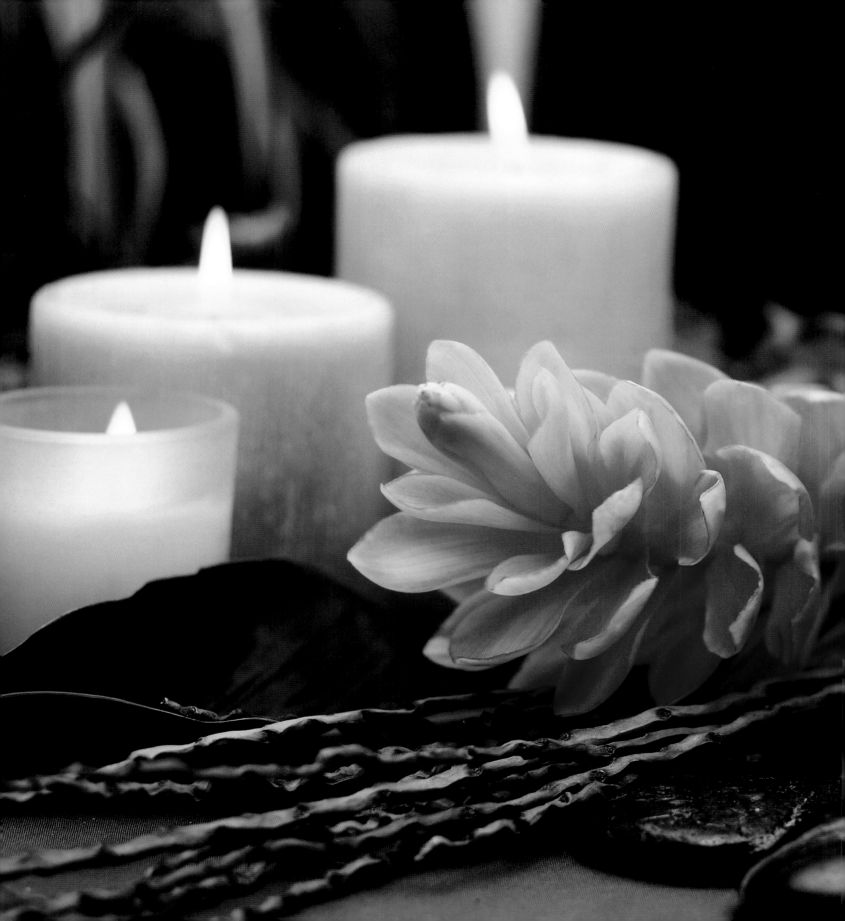

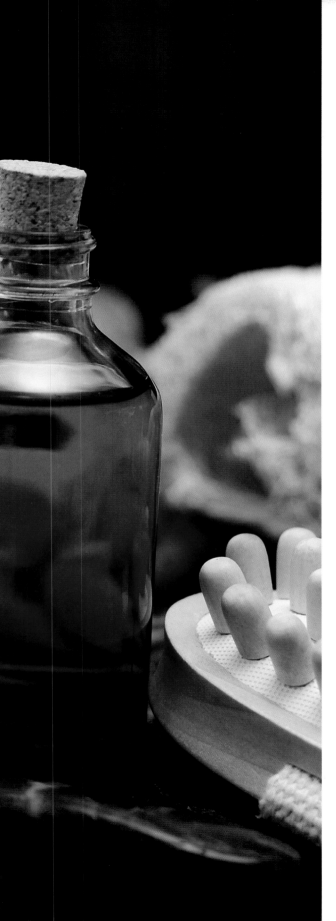

LEFT: Essential oils stimulate the sense of smell, which has been shown to elicit the strongest emotional reactions.

Now relax, breathe slowly and deeply, and enjoy the sense of nurturing, caring, and compassion that's conveyed through every touch.

HEALING WITH SMELL: AROMATHERAPY

Basil to uplift, lemon to refresh, lavender to calm—inhaling the fragrances of such common herbs, fruits, and flowers can dramatically affect how we think and feel. When we inhale a scent, olfactory nerve cells send the information to the limbic system of the brain, which is associated with memory, mood, and emotions. The sense of smell has a direct connection to this part of the brain.

Smell bypasses the nervous system; thus, when we smell something it can prompt an immediate reaction—physiological or psychological, positive or negative. Research has shown that of the five senses, smell elicits the strongest emotional responses. Just one aroma—perhaps cinnamon buns baking—can stir up vivid images from our childhood even though decades may have passed.

Humans can distinguish an infinite number of smells, each of which contains chemical compounds that influence in different ways. For example, chamomile, frankincense, and sandalwood sedate; bay leaf, rosemary, and ginger stimulate.

Papyri dating back to the reign of the Egyptian pharaoh Khufu in the twenty-sixth century BC tell of aristocrats who used fragrant resins and barks for medicinal and cosmetic purposes. These materials also were burned as incense during rituals; the resultant smoke, it was believed, lifted their prayers to heaven. "Perfume" is derived from the Latin words *per* (through) and *fumus* (smoke).

BELOW: Chamomile is brewed into a tea that helps ease stress and anxiety.

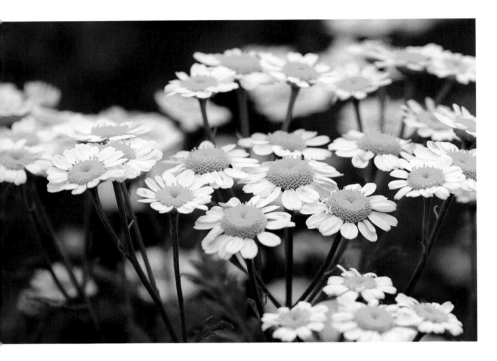

Modern health practitioners agree aromatherapy makes good "scents." As Gattefosse found, essential oils can either be inhaled or absorbed through the skin to obtain physiological benefits. These range from relieving fluid retention; soothing cuts; and reducing aches, stiffness, and inflammation to staving off colds and coughs; easing nausea and indigestion; and diminishing the signs of acne, eczema, and ringworm.

Among the most popular essential oils are bergamot, chamomile, clary sage, cypress, eucalyptus, frankincense, geranium, grapefruit, jasmine absolute, juniper, lavender, lemon, marjoram, neroli, patchouli, peppermint, rose, rosemary, sandalwood, sweet orange, tea tree, vetiver, and ylang-ylang. Because pure essential oils are very concentrated, they always should be diluted with a "carrier oil" before being applied to the skin.

Common carrier oils include apricot kernel, avocado, grape seed, jojoba, olive, rose hip, safflower, sweet almond, sunflower, and wheat germ. Many Hawaiian blends contain coconut, *kukui* (candlenut), or macadamia nut as carrier oils.

Even though these oils are "natural," they should be used with care. Some may cause redness, itching, or other skin irritations, so it's a good idea to do a patch test of diluted essential oil on the inside of your wrist or in the crease of your elbow when trying it for the first time. Wait twenty-four hours to see if you have a reaction.

Other tips:

• Find a reputable supplier to ensure you're getting "pure" essential oils, not synthetic chemicals. Be sure your choices have been filled to the top of small, dark glass bottles with droppers built into the opening so

The process of distillation to extract plants' essential oils was not discovered until the late tenth century, presumably by an Arab physician and alchemist named Avicenna. French chemist Rene-Maurice Gattefosse coined the word "aromatherapy"—the use of essential oils for health benefits—in the early 1930s. As the story goes, he was working on an experiment in his laboratory one day when an explosion seriously injured his hand. He dipped his hand into a bowl of pure lavender oil that happened to be resting on a nearby countertop.

That not only brought immediate relief, it enabled the burn to heal very quickly with no infection or scarring. Intrigued, Gattefosse began investigating the therapeutic properties of essential oils, and published his findings in a groundbreaking 1937 book entitled *Aromatherapie.*

BELOW: Essential oils can either be inhaled or absorbed through the skin to provide a host of psychological and physiological benefits.

when you turn the bottle upside down, one drop at a time is released. Never use plastic bottles; plastic is porous and will allow the oils to escape and evaporate.

• Because the quality of essential oils deteriorates in heat and light, they should be stored in a cool, dark place (never in extreme temperatures—that is, neither freezing nor above ninety-five degrees). To prevent evaporation, be sure the lids are tightly closed. Most essential oils will keep this way for about two years (label the bottles with the names of the oils and the dates you purchased them). Once they have been blended with a carrier oil, however, they'll only be good for a few months.

• You can prolong the life of essential oils by storing them in the refrigerator. The bottle lids should be secured tightly so the aromas do not permeate food. Oils that have a high wax content may solidify when refrigerated, but will liquefy when brought back to room temperature.

• The color of the oils may change over time. Don't worry; this won't affect their potency.

• Essential oils are flammable, so don't expose them to open flames. Also keep them out of reach of children and pets, as they can be toxic if ingested in large amounts.

• Essential oils can mar polished surfaces. Be sure you clean up spills right away.

• As you make your blends, carefully dispense the essential oils by the drop. (It is imperative that you use a dropper so you can carefully control amounts.) Since the oils are very concentrated, they should be used sparingly. When in doubt, use less rather than more.

• Do not apply essential oils around your eyes. If they accidentally get in your eyes, rinse immediately with cool water.

• Never use essential oils internally unless you've been advised to do so by your doctor or a qualified aromatherapist.

• Be aware of contraindications. For example, epileptics shouldn't use stimulants such as sage and fennel. Expectant mothers should avoid certain essential oils, including basil, hyssop, and myrrh. In general, oils that are safe to use during pregnancy come from flowers—rose, ylang-ylang, jasmine, lavender, and the like. Other oils are phototoxic, meaning they can damage your skin if you're exposed to sunlight after using them. Bergamot, for example, contains a phototoxic chemical called bergatene, so any bergamot purchased should be NS (nonsensitizing) or BF (bergatene free), meaning the chemical has been removed. Citrus oils also tend to be phototoxic. When in doubt, consult your doctor to find out which oils are safe for you.

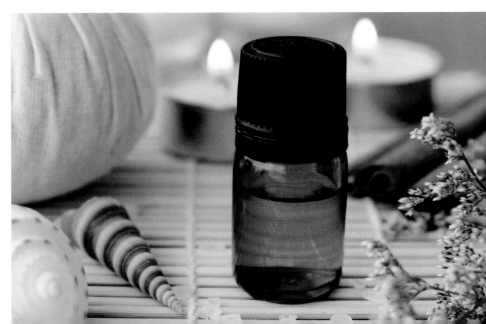

BELOW: At Aveda Lifestyle Salon & Spa on O'ahu, you can create your own shampoo, conditioner, massage oil, and cleansing formula from sixteen preblended oils.

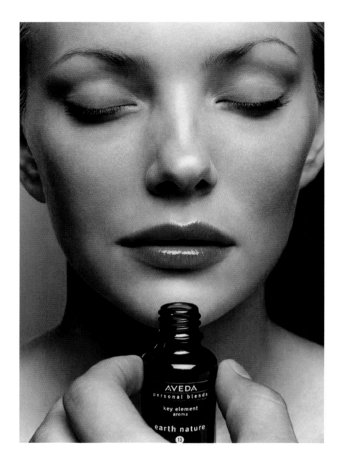

• Essential oils also can alleviate emotional problems such as anxiety, insomnia, and depression. During the Aveda Sensory Journey at Aveda Lifestyle Salon & Spa at Ala Moana Center, you'll select from sixteen preblended oils that will provide the result you seek, whether it be to energize, refresh, calm, or balance. Purchase an aroma-neutral body- or hair-care base—such as a shampoo, conditioner, massage oil, or cleansing formula—and, with the help of an Aveda "aroma-ology" adviser, create your own unique product using the oils you chose. This service is free.

The following bath and massage oil recipes are provided courtesy of Aveda Corporation. For baths, add one or two drops of essential oil to a tub filled with warm water. You can use just one essential oil or blend the aromas in the recipes—as long as a total of no more than two drops are added to the tub. Add the oils just before you enter the bath so they don't dissipate in the steam. Be sure to mix them into the water well so they don't settle in one spot and irritate your skin (remember, they are concentrated substances).

The recommended dilution for body massage oils is 1 percent, or ten drops of essential oil (or essential oil blend) per ounce (two tablespoons) of carrier oil. If you wish to blend oils for use on the face, use a 0.5 percent dilution, or five drops per ounce (less if you have sensitive skin). You also can place a teaspoon to a tablespoon of massage oil in a bath.

To Uplift or Improve a Sad Mood
Blend 1: 7 drops clary sage, 3 drops grapefruit
Blend 2: 8 drops lavender, 2 drops jasmine absolute
Blend 3: 5 drops lemon, 5 drops orange
Bath: lavender, neroli, jasmine absolute, clary sage

To Sharpen Memory and Concentration
Blend 1: 5 drops rosemary, 5 drops lavender
Blend 2: 8 drops bergamot, 2 drops peppermint
Blend 3: 6 drops eucalyptus, 4 drops cypress
Bath: rosemary (no more than 1 drop), lavender, tea tree, eucalyptus

To Energize, Refresh, and Stimulate
Blend 1: 5 drops juniper, 5 drops marjoram
Blend 2: 7 drops tea tree, 3 drops peppermint
Blend 3: 7 drops rosemary, 3 drops marjoram
Bath: tea tree, bergamot, marjoram

To Relieve Stress and Anxiety

Blend 1: 8 drops bergamot, 2 drops lavender
Blend 2: 6 drops patchouli, 4 drops frankincense
Blend 3: 9 drops bergamot, 1 drop rose
Bath: rose, clary sage, bergamot

To Relieve Insomnia

Blend 1: 6 drops chamomile, 4 drops lavender
Blend 2: 6 drops vetiver, 4 drops ylang-ylang
Blend 3: 7 drops lavender, 3 drops sandalwood
Bath: lavender, chamomile, vetiver, sandalwood

To Relieve Depression

Blend 1: 6 drops clary sage, 4 drops frankincense
Blend 2: 7 drops geranium, 3 drops neroli
Blend 3: 8 drops ylang-ylang, 2 drops rose
Bath: clary sage, neroli, rose, ylang-ylang

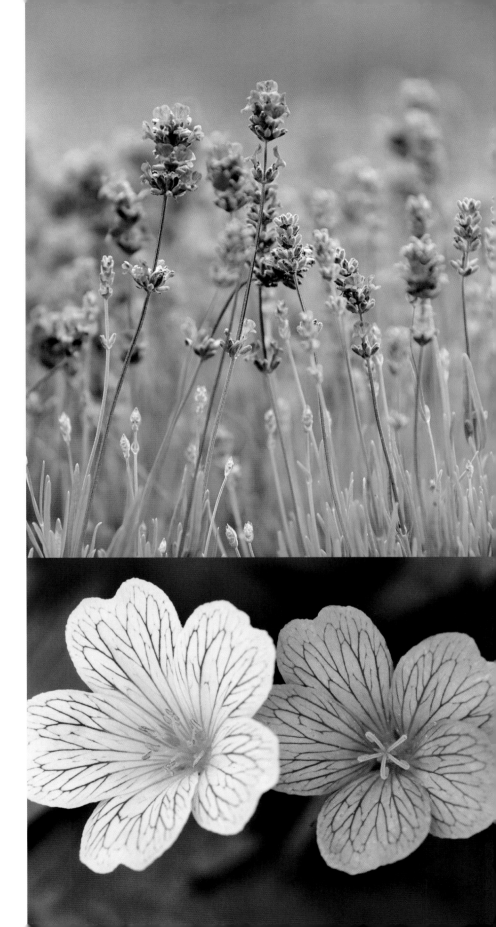

TOP RIGHT: The scent of lavender can balance you; for example, rejuvenate you if you're tired and relax you if you're uptight.

BOTTOM RIGHT: Aromatherapists use essential oil distilled from geraniums for numerous ailments, including arthritis and asthma.

HEALING WITH SIGHT: COLOR THERAPY

Chromotherapy, the use of color as a healing agent, dates back over three thousand years to the time of the ancient Egyptians. In the temple in the city of Heliopolis, which was the center of worship for the sun god Ra, sunlight was refracted into the colors of the rainbow—red, orange, yellow, green, blue, indigo, and violet—and directed into seven different chambers. There, patients absorbed the warmth and color of the brilliant rays through their skin and eyes, as they believed that provided a multitude of therapeutic benefits.

Long ago in Russia, covering a patient with a red flannel blanket was considered to be an effective remedy for scarlet fever. Red wool wrappings were used to treat sprains in Scotland; and in Portugal, wearing a piece of red coral supposedly relieved headaches. In Japan during the early nineteenth century, when the children of the emperor contracted smallpox, they were confined in a room filled with red furnishings, which supposedly accelerated the healing process.

Yellow was used to combat jaundice. In olden England, eating yellow spiders rolled in butter was thought to be the best cure for the disease; in Germany, yellow turnips and saffron were consumed for the same reason.

The Irish tied blue ribbons around their throats to battle croup and green thread around their waists to ease indigestion. Blue and green also were worn as preventives to ward off sickness.

While some may regard all this as little more than old wives' tales, studies have shown color can indeed produce profound psychological and physiological reactions. Here's how it works: Color is a phenomenon of light, which is composed of electromagnetic waves of energy. When light hits the retina, it is converted into chemical and nervous signals, which travel to the brain and prompt the release of hormones—molecular "messengers" that, in turn, trigger responses in other parts of the body.

It is well known that throughout the bleak winters of northern climates, Seasonal Affective Disorder (SAD) is a common complaint. Symptoms include depression, irritability, lack of energy, oversleeping, overeating, and weight gain. SAD has been linked to the sleep-promoting hormone melatonin, which is produced at higher levels when it's dark. Exposing people with SAD to full-spectrum light from a bright light box (deemed the closest simulation to natural sunlight) lowered their daytime levels of melatonin, which has depressive effects, and raised the amount of the mood-elevating brain chemical serotonin.

Chromopaths, practitioners of color therapy, reason that if light and the absence of it have major effects on health, then the colors that make up light must follow suit. Like food, they explain, color supplies energy to the body. All vital organs are directly connected to the skin via the arteries, capillaries, and blood vessels. Applying color to a problem area theoretically draws blood to it, increasing circulation and eliminating toxins, thus promoting healing.

In addition, they point out that iron, zinc, sodium, magnesium, and other key life-sustaining elements can be taken into the body either by consuming foods or by being absorbed through exposure. Sunlight, for example, is a significant source of vitamin D.

Applications of color therapy vary widely, from soaking in colored baths and focusing beams of colored light on ailing parts of the body to visualizing a particular color while meditating and wearing clothes or eating foods of recommended colors.

Each color has different effects. For example:

RED energizes and excites. It pumps up the metabolism and muscular system, increases heart rate, improves circulation, and heightens the senses. It counteracts depression, anemia, low blood pressure, and lethargy. It is the color of vitality and strength, but prolonged exposure may induce fever, anxiety, or aggression.

BLUE soothes and calms. It relaxes muscles, fights inflammation, promotes sleep, and reduces heart rate and high blood pressure. It relieves pain, stress, fever, headache, burns, insomnia, and infection. It is the color of coolness and serenity, but prolonged exposure can result in fatigue, sorrow, or melancholia.

YELLOW stimulates and uplifts. It aids concentration, sharpens mental ability, and activates the motor nerves. It treats rheumatism, arthritis, constipation, depression, and digestive problems, and promotes confidence, optimism, and *joie de vivre*. It is the color of intellect and clarity, but prolonged exposure can bring on hyperactivity or insomnia.

GREEN balances and refreshes. It lowers blood pressure, quiets the nervous system, and stabilizes emotions. It combats irritability, tension, exhaustion, ulcers, and headaches, and is regarded as a healing, sedating force. It is the color of harmony and growth, but prolonged exposure can be tiring or arouse negative feelings.

PURPLE purifies and comforts. It eases pain, lowers blood pressure, and has narcotic and hypnotic effects. It is beneficial for rheumatism, epilepsy, headaches, stiffness, cysts, and mental and nervous problems. It is the color of royalty and dignity, but prolonged exposure can suppress emotions (especially anger) or contribute to depression.

ORANGE cheers and invigorates. It regulates circulation and metabolism, and encourages a sense of well-being and sociableness. It alleviates depression, asthma, bronchitis, indigestion, and muscle spasms and cramps. It is the color of joy and creativity, but prolonged exposure can make you feel nervous or agitated.

Although there are those who tout the success of chromotherapy with serious diseases such as AIDS, cancer, and diabetes, it only should be used as an adjunct to the medical treatment prescribed by a physician.

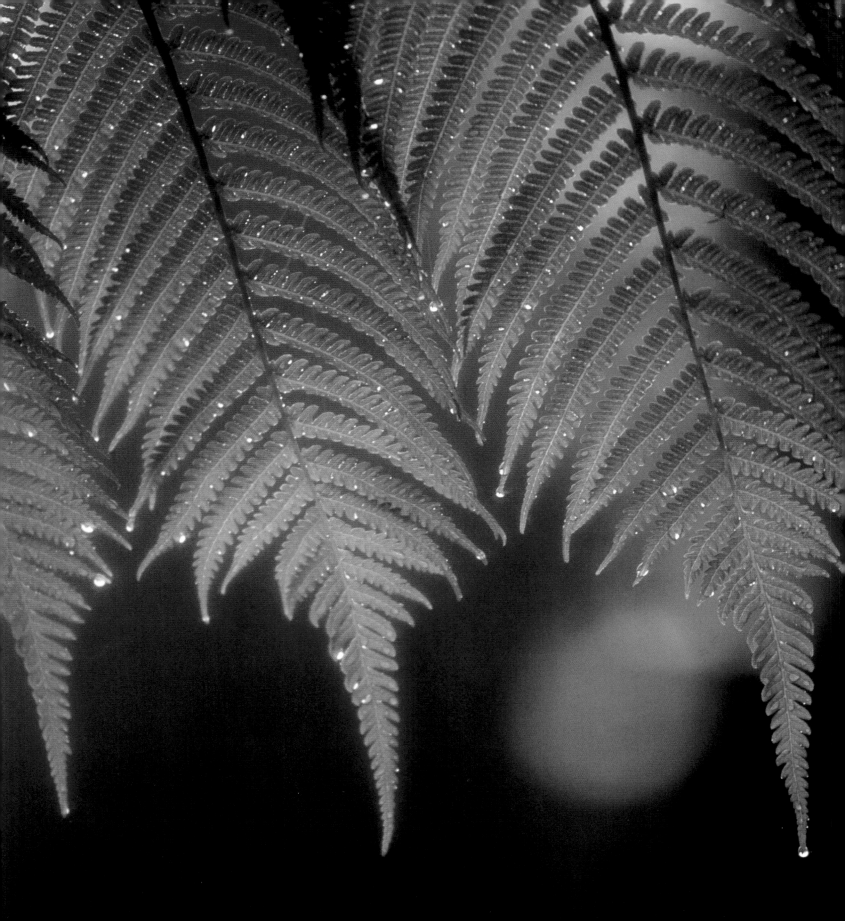

LEFT: Soft, harmonious sounds like rainfall can put you in a peaceful, meditative mood.

HEALING WITH SOUND: MUSIC THERAPY

There's no question that sound plays a significant role in our lives. We communicate, learn, relax, get motivated, and are alerted to danger through sound. We wake up to sound; play and work to sound; and unwind at night to sound from the radio, the TV, or a CD. We remember the lullabies that soothed us to sleep as children, the hits we listened to when we hung out with friends in our youth, the songs that symbolized our love when we married. We know what we like to hear when we eat, read, exercise, and socialize.

It's no wonder, then, that sound is becoming increasingly popular as a complementary therapeutic measure to get one's entire being "in tune." This therapy is based on the premise that sound travels in waves of energy whose variables—including velocity, frequency, and intensity—give each sound its unique characteristics. The ear processes these waves and sends impulses to the brain, which produces definite responses.

For instance, when we're exposed to loud, prolonged, discordant sounds, our blood pressure rises, blood vessels constrict, muscles tighten, and pulse rate quickens—signs of stress that place added burden on the heart. Being subjected to continual noise also has been linked to headache, fatigue, ulcers, and loss of hearing.

On the other hand, soft, harmonious sounds are mood enhancers. They calm, alleviate pain, and reduce tension and anxiety. When we're awake, our brain operates on a beta wave frequency. Gentle sound therapy moves it into the deeper alpha and theta wave frequencies that prevail when we're peaceful, relaxed, and meditative— the state that's most conducive to healing.

An old Greek saying observes: "Men have song as a physician for pain." History shows this indeed seems to be the case. Since the dawn of civilization, shamans and mystics around the globe have used drums, maracas, and other percussion instruments to heal the sick. The Chinese *I Ching* (Book of Changes), written some five thousand years ago, is one of the oldest and most famous books on philosophy, divination, cosmology, and personal enlightenment in the world. It asserts, "Music has the power to ease tension within the heart, and to lessen and loosen obscure emotions."

Egyptian papyri dating back twenty-six hundred years speak of incantations to cure infertility, rheumatism, and other complaints. According to the Phoenician-born philosopher Porphyry (AD 233 to 305), the renowned Greek philosopher and mathematician Pythagoras (580 to 500 BC) recognized music's ability to exert "a healing, purifying influence on human actions and passions, restoring the pristine harmony of the soul's faculties." In the Bible, the young shepherd David calmed the manic moods of King Saul with melodic tunes on his harp.

Music—valued for its accessibility, affordability, effectiveness, safety, and ease of use—is the most common of contemporary sound therapies. Options range from singing, chanting, and playing instruments to writing tunes, combining music and imagery, and humming and toning (elongating a sound using the breath and voice). The most popular method is simply listening to a "prescription" of music for a predetermined period, usually thirty minutes to a few hours a day for at least a month.

Violin, piano, flute, guitar, Tibetan singing bowls, tuning forks, gongs, bells, chimes—the sounds for music therapy come from many sources, both familiar and uncommon. Nature also offers a vast repertoire of voices that lull us into relaxation, including the rustle of leaves, the warble of birds, the songs of whales and dolphins, the crackle of a campfire, the ebb and flow of waves, and the pitter-patter of rain.

Harmonic music with an even tempo and pleasant timbre (for example, string instruments as opposed to brass) seems to work best for most people. In addition, the rhythm should be slow and steady, containing about seventy to eighty beats per minute, in cadence with the heartbeat. A faster cadence may stimulate the body to the point of inducing stress, nervousness, and apprehension. Also, the music should be low in pitch and volume; high pitch and volume also may cause tension.

Instrumental selections are preferable to those with vocals because the mind will tend to focus on the words of the latter rather than wind down to the music. Baroque, new age, Gregorian chant, and classical are excellent choices—particularly, research has shown, the music of Mozart.

For optimum results, remove all jewelry and wear loose clothing for your session. Lie on a comfortable flat surface such as a bed, or sit in a cozy chair with your legs and arms uncrossed. The temperature of the room should be warm, but there should be a window open so fresh air can circulate. As the music plays, keep your eyes closed and continue to breathe deeply.

Regular doses of "music medicine" have proven beneficial in many ways, including reducing heart rate, blood pressure, and muscle tension; alleviating pain, fatigue, digestive problems, and depression; facilitating movement and childbirth; promoting relaxation and sleep; and improving mood, concentration, and learning abilities. Most people think music is only for the ears, but that's not true. With music therapy, the whole body listens.

HEALING WITH TASTE: SPA CUISINE

Spa cuisine is healthy cuisine, but that doesn't mean limited choices and bland preparations. Using fresh, wholesome foods that have been minimally processed, spa chefs are creating innovative, delicious, satisfying dishes that would win compliments from even the most finicky gourmet.

Ingredients for spa cuisine are high in antioxidants, vitamins, and minerals, and low in fat; sodium; cholesterol; sugar; "empty" calories; and artificial sweeteners, preservatives, and colorings. These include whole grains, legumes, lentils, and beans; fresh fruits and vegetables; protein, primarily tofu and lean meats; nonfat dairy products; herbs, spices, vinegars, and oils for seasonings; and liberal amounts of omega-3 fatty acids (good sources are albacore tuna, mackerel, trout, herring, sardines, and salmon).

Preferred cooking methods are boiling, broiling, poaching, steaming, grilling, and roasting. Rich sauces, gravies, and coatings are shunned. Instead, simple presentations enhance the natural beauty, flavor, texture, and nutritional value of the food. Portions are sensible, and meals are balanced—even including healthy sweets such as apricot mousse whipped up with nonfat cottage cheese and nonfat yogurt, and applesauce cookies made with egg whites, whole wheat flour, and unsweetened apple juice and applesauce.

Cookbooks from acclaimed American spas offer delicious and healthy recipes, including:

Adventure Cuisine Cookbook
Red Mountain Spa
www.redmountainspa.com

Cal-a-Vie's Gourmet Spa Cookery
Cal-a-Vie
www.calavie.com

Canyon Ranch Cooks: Great Tastes
Canyon Ranch Cooks: More
 Great Tastes
Canyon Ranch Cooks: More Than
 200 Delicious, Innovative
 Recipes from America's Leading
 Health Resort
Canyon Ranch
www.canyonranch.com

Deerfield Spa's Casual Cooking
Deerfield Spa
www.deerfieldspa.com

Fresh: Healthy Cooking and Living
 from Lake Austin Spa Resort
Lean Star Cuisine
Lake Austin Spa Resort
www.lakeaustin.com

The Golden Door Cooks Light
 and Easy
Golden Door
www.goldendoor.com

The Green Valley Cookbook
Green Valley Spa and Resort
www.greenvalleyspa.com

Healthy Cooking for Singles
 and Doubles
Recipes for Fitness for Very Busy People
Newest Favorite Recipes for Fitness
 from The Oaks at Ojai
The Ultimate Recipe for Fitness: Spa
 Cuisine from The Oaks at Ojai
 and the Palms at Palm Springs
The Oaks at Ojai
www.oaksspa.com

The Heartland Spa Recipe
 Collection
The Heartland Spa
www.heartlandspa.com

The Kerr House Cookbook: A
 Treasury of Recipes for Mind,
 Body and Soul
The Kerr House
www.thekerrhouse.com

Our Favorite Recipes
New Favorites
Tennessee Fitness Spa
www.tfspa.com

Recipes for Living
Green Mountain at Fox Run
www.fitwoman.com

The Shoshoni Cookbook:
 Vegetarian Recipes from
 the Shoshoni Yoga Retreat
Shoshoni Yoga Retreat
www.shoshoni.org

The Six Senses Cookbook
Six Senses Resorts & Spas
www.sixsenses.com

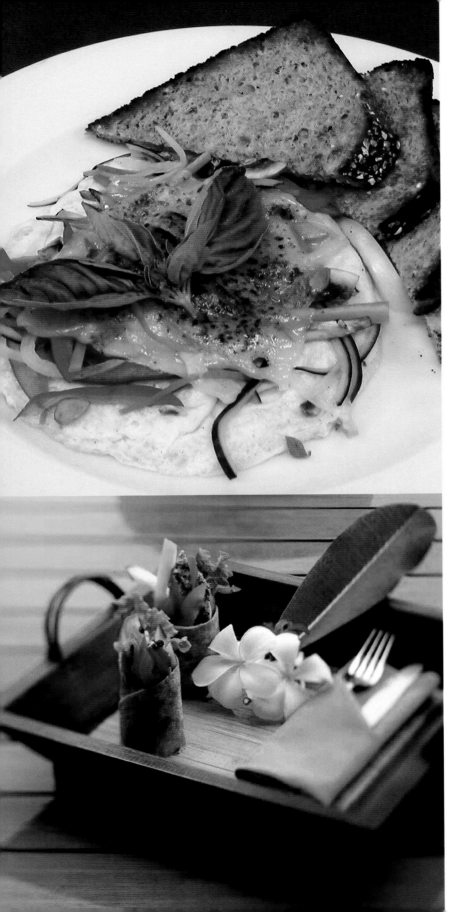

TOP LEFT: The Kohala Spa Omelet is a healthy, delicious combination of egg whites, low-fat cheese, and fresh vegetables.

BOTTOM LEFT: You can make the pretty, nutritious Da Wrap in minutes.

Recipes

Kohala Spa Omelet

Courtesy of Hilton Waikoloa Village, Island of Hawai'i

3	egg whites
1	Tbsp. each of bell pepper, red onion, white onion, carrots, mushrooms, marinated tomatoes, broccoli and asparagus, julienned
¼	c. Swiss or low-fat cheese, shredded
½	c. low-fat yogurt
¼	c. fresh honeydew, strawberries, and cantaloupe

Cook egg whites in a sauté pan, at the same time steaming vegetables for 30 seconds in a separate pot. Place the steamed vegetables on the cooked eggs. Put cheese on the vegetables (it will melt). Transfer omelet to plate, garnish with yogurt and fruits, and serve with toast and fruit preserves. Serves 1.

Da Wrap

Courtesy of Kūpono Café, Anara Spa, Grand Hyatt Kaua'i Resort & Spa, Kaua'i

2	Tbsp. Cilantro and Sun-Dried Tomato Spread
1	spinach tortilla
2½	oz. turkey or chicken
2	leaves baby red leaf lettuce
2	tomatoes, sliced
2	slices (2 oz.) pre-sliced cheese, either Swiss, provolone, or cheddar
⅓	yellow pepper, julienned
¼	c. sunflower sprouts

Spread Cilantro and Sun-Dried Tomato Spread on spinach tortilla. Add meat, lettuce, tomato, cheese, yellow pepper, and sprouts. Roll into tube shape, then cut in half. Serves 1.

Cilantro and Sun-Dried Tomato Spread

2   Tbsp. fat-free cream cheese (room temperature)
1   Tbsp. fat-free sour cream
2   tsp. sun-dried tomato (reconstituted with warm water, then pureed)
1   tsp. cilantro, chopped
½   tsp. lime juice
Salt to taste
Pepper to taste

Mix all ingredients. Add salt and pepper according to your preference.

Miso-Glazed Salmon

Courtesy of Ihilani Spa, JW Marriott Ihilani Resort & Spa, O'ahu

1   bunch baby bok choy or other local greens such as chard, choy sum, or won bok
⅓   stalk lemongrass (lower portion), crushed
2   whole fresh shiitake mushrooms
2   Tbsp. fresh corn kernels
Pinch salt
Pinch sugar
½   lb. salmon steak
Pinch miso paste
1   tsp. chopped red bell pepper
1   tsp. shaved or finely chopped green onions
2   lemongrass spears (upper portion)

Preheat oven to 400 degrees. Blanch bok choy in salted boiling water. Remove when cooked and refresh in ice water. Drain and set aside until ready to serve. Make a broth by simmering lemongrass stalk with mushrooms, corn kernels, salt, and sugar until corn and mushrooms are tender. Strain out corn and mushrooms, and set aside. Place simmered liquid in a pan to reduce slowly while baking salmon. Brush salmon with miso paste and bake for 10 to 15 minutes, until just cooked (do not overcook, as it will become dry). Place bok choy in the middle of a large soup plate and put the salmon on top of it. Pour the reduced lemongrass broth over the salmon, then spoon the mushrooms and corn relish on it. Garnish with chopped red pepper and green onions. Top with lemongrass spears placed like an X. Serves 1.

HEALING WITH THE MIND: MEDITATION

Say the word "meditation" and Benedictine monks may come to mind, but today, of course, meditation isn't a discipline you only find in remote monasteries. It's an essential part of an integrated health program that's safe and simple to do.

Countless studies have proven the power of the mind. Meditation can alleviate anxiety, depression, and irritability. It can increase creativity, vitality, and equanimity; enhance learning and problem-solving abilities; and awaken feelings of hope and happiness. It can help you get grounded, cope with pain and stress, and develop inner peace and a positive outlook on life.

Meditation also has been shown to improve circulation and the flow of oxygen to the lungs; slow the metabolism and heart rate; decrease blood pressure, respiration, muscle tension, and levels of cortisol and lactate (two chemicals associated with stress); and reduce free radicals, which, because of the damage they can wreak on cells and tissues, are regarded as a major factor in aging and many diseases. Collectively, these changes induce a "relaxation response"—an aid in the healing process.

The use of meditation to treat illness is not a new concept; rooted in religion, it has been practiced by diverse cultures around the world for thousands of years. There are many forms of meditation, but they have one common intent: to subdue an active mind. Most techniques consist of four basic components:

A quiet place. Choose a spot with minimal noise, interruptions, and distractions. Burn incense or set out a bowl of potpourri or a vase of fresh flowers to scent the room. Play soft music.

An erect, comfortable posture. Sitting on the floor is better than lying down because you don't want to risk going to sleep. Keep your spine straight, clasp your hands, cross your legs, and close your eyes. (If you're unable to sit cross-legged on the floor, you can sit erect in a chair, with both feet on the floor.) You should be still and relaxed, but alert.

Point of focus. This could be a neutral word; a mantra such as "Oommmm"; even your own slow, deep, regular breathing. It's best to select something that won't stir up long trains of associated thoughts, since the purpose of meditation is to quiet the mind. Acknowledge any feelings, images, memories, and sensations that may arise without reacting to them.

Relaxed awareness. Relaxation and alertness should be in balance; you should be able to release all the tension in your body and view all distractions with complete detachment. If you start responding to something, bring your attention back to your chosen focus. Gently clear the clutter from your brain, and complete restfulness will be your reward. When your session is done, preserve this feeling by not bounding back into reality. Sit quietly for a minute or so, keeping your eyes closed. Then open your eyes, but continue sitting for another few minutes before going on with your day.

Visualization is another effective relaxation technique; you might describe it as daydreaming with a purpose. Simply put, you usher yourself to a serene state by conjuring up pleasurable thoughts. For instance, imagine you're in a tranquil meadow. Fragrant wildflowers are sprouting up everywhere, cool breezes are playing with your hair, and horses are contentedly grazing nearby. You're sitting beside a gurgling brook, munching on a crisp, sweet apple. Immerse yourself in the setting, making note of every wonderful sight, sound, smell, taste, and feeling.

Or picture a big, empty box. One by one, put everything that is bothering you into that box. Cover it and move it to the side. Relaxing shouldn't be difficult now that your problems are out of the way. Similarly, you can dig a large hole in your mind and "bury" your troubles there.

During guided imagery, a person with a soothing voice helps draw a place in your mind with broad strokes. You paint the suggested scene with appealing details; for instance, you not only see a beautiful beach, but you smell the salt-laden air, hear the rush of the waves, touch the soft sand, and feel the warmth of the sun. Your body should respond favorably to this construct as if it were real.

If possible, reserve twenty to thirty minutes at the same time each day for meditation (before breakfast is ideal). No matter what technique you choose, it's important that you be mindful—that is, that you linger "in the moment." Don't worry about things that happened in the past or what's on your list of things to do. "Now" is all that matters.

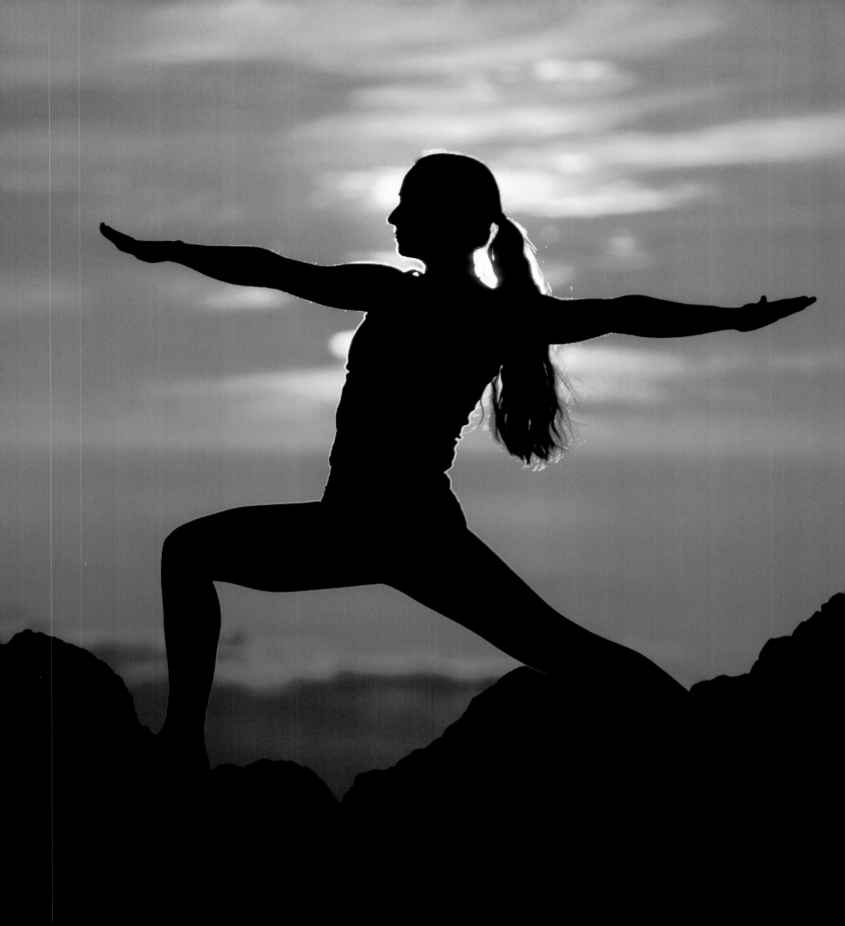

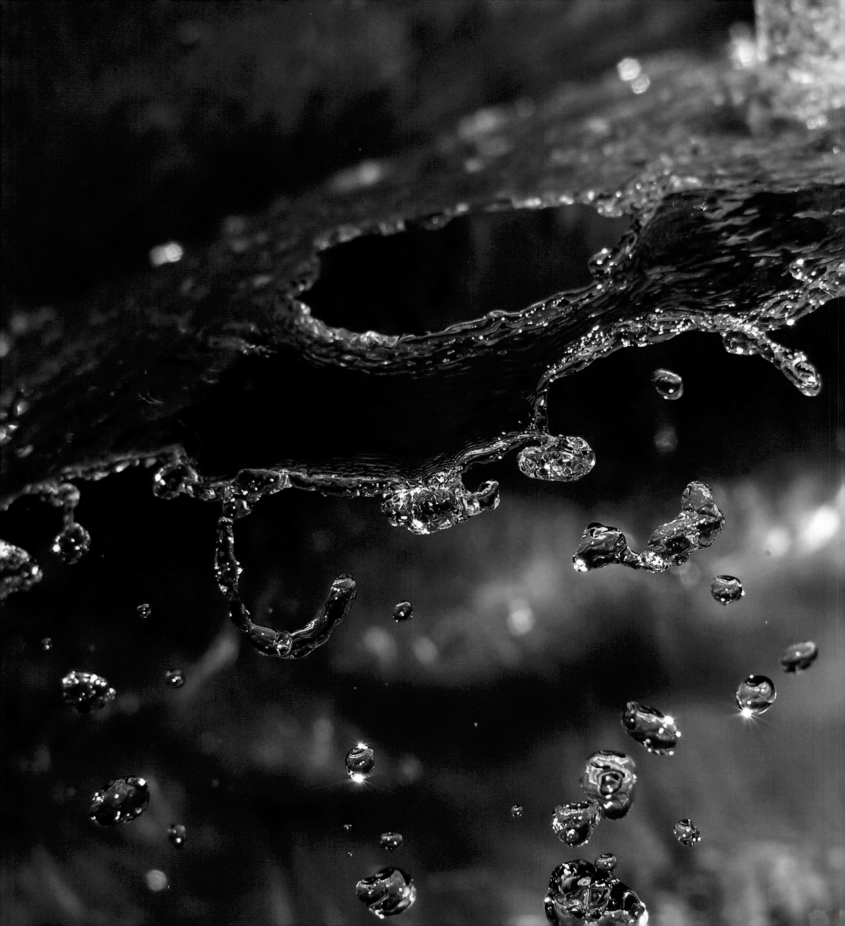

LEFT: Baths, whirlpool soaks, aqua bodywork, and other forms of hydrotherapy prove water is an effective healing agent.

HEALING WITH WATER: HYDROTHERAPY

Water is essential to survival. We can live without food for several weeks, but only three to six days without water. In fact, about 60 percent of the adult human body is composed of water. Without adequate water in our system, blood does not circulate properly, toxins can't be expelled, organ tissues deteriorate, and other vital physiological processes are disrupted.

Because of that, many health experts believe dehydration leads to disease. They suggest headache, heartburn, arthritis, asthma, indigestion, fatigue, back pain, hypertension, and other common ailments can be prevented and possibly cured by increasing the intake of pure water. On average, adults should drink at least two quarts of water each day. Doing this is one of the biggest steps you can take toward good health.

Called hydrotherapy, water also can be used externally as a solid, liquid, or vapor to promote well-being. Because it is readily available, inexpensive, and an excellent conductor of heat and cold, water is a popular and effective therapeutic agent.

Hydrotherapy dates back eons, the famed baths of Rome being among its most elaborate examples. For the upper class at the height of the Roman Empire, bathing was a daily ritual that went on for at least a few hours in lavish establishments called *thermae*. Reminiscent of modern spas and health clubs, these public facilities encompassed gardens, libraries, promenades, shops, hair salons, theaters, and gymnasiums as well as baths. Many *thermae* reflected the opulence of palaces, with mirrored walls, high vaulted ceilings, marble-lined pools, intricate floor mosaics, beautiful paintings, and silver faucets.

Today, we consider bathing to be very much a private practice, but the baths of ancient Rome were popular social spots where conversation ranged from friendly chitchat to serious business discussions. Bathers moved leisurely through various areas, including the *tepidarium*, with heated walls and floors; the *calidarium*, with large soaking tubs filled with hot water; and the *frigidarium*, with a cold pool.

Instead of water, wealthy patrons often enjoyed a bath in wine or milk followed by a massage with perfumes scented with resins, bark, and flowers. They then attended lectures, watched athletic competitions and performances by jugglers and acrobats, bought tasty tidbits from an assortment of food vendors, or strolled in the luxurious environs. In AD 305, the emperor Diocletian oversaw the construction of a magnificent thirty-two-acre *thermae* that could accommodate three thousand bathers. By the end of the fourth century, there were over nine hundred bathhouses in Rome.

Modern health practitioners hail the therapeutic properties of baths, especially those in thermal springs. They believe these natural hot pools promote healing in several ways, including releasing toxins; easing muscle stiffness; aiding digestion; mending wounds; promoting relaxation and production of painkilling endorphins; alleviating skin conditions such as psoriasis and fungal infections; and increasing metabolism, blood flow, and oxygenation of cells.

Other forms of hydrotherapy include sitz baths, ice packs, hand baths and footbaths, hot and cold compresses, whirlpool soaks, steam inhalations, steam and sauna rooms, flotation, thalassotherapy, Scotch hose massage, Swiss and Vichy showers, and aqua bodywork such as Watsu (definitions of the latter six can be found in the glossary).

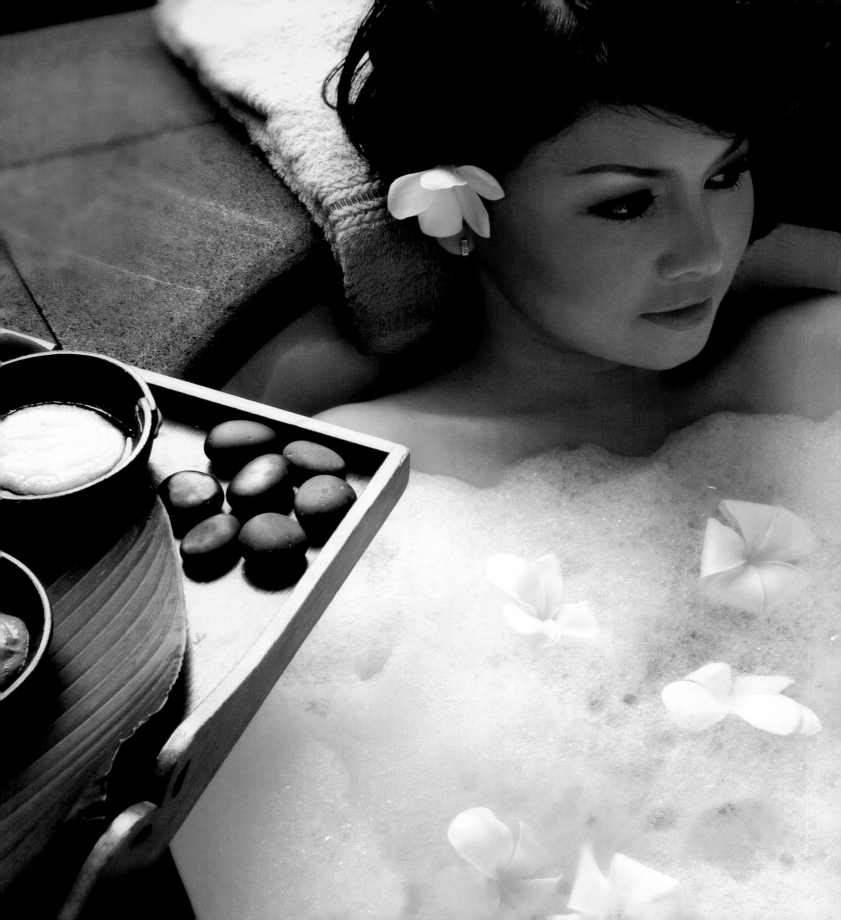

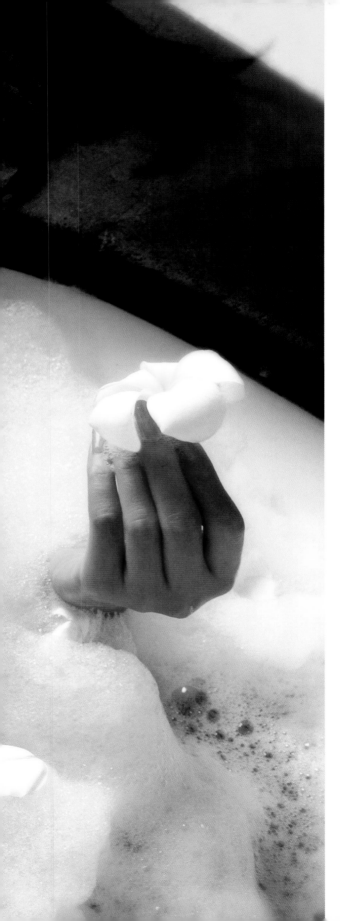

LEFT: A warm,
leisurely bath is
a great way to
reduce tension.

There are cautions about hydrotherapy that should be
noted, however, including:

• Extreme hot and cold temperatures are not recommended if you have disorders such as a heart problem,
lung disease, diabetes, a kidney infection, high or low
blood pressure, or an infectious skin condition. In general, temperatures ranging too high or too low from the
normal body temperature of 98.6 can injure the skin and
tissues.

• Don't soak in thermal springs if you have a skin
disease or are under the influence of alcohol or drugs,
especially heart medications.

• Don't heat a compress in the microwave because it
will get too hot too quickly. Instead, soak it in hot water
from the tap and test the temperature before applying it
to your skin.

• When you use a pot of boiling water for steam inhalation, be sure you take it off the stove to cool a bit first.
There should be no active boiling when you inhale, as
that can scald your face and respiratory tract. Keep your
face about a foot away from the pot and cover your
head and shoulders with a towel so the steam won't
escape before you can breathe it.

• Be aware that cold hydrotherapy options such as ice
packs and cold compresses constrict blood vessels,
numb nerves, and slow respiration. Warm and hot therapies such as whirlpools and thermal springs produce the
opposite effect.

• Icing a sprain, strain, or bruise that isn't too severe will
minimize swelling and internal bleeding, but be sure
that you wrap the ice in a towel before applying it, as
direct contact with your skin can cause nerve damage.

• Cold compresses can ease the pain of gout and swelling from bruises and sprains, but limit applications to twenty minutes at a time so you won't damage your skin.

• Don't eat a heavy meal before bathing; the best time to bathe is when you have an empty stomach.

• Some people feel light-headed when soaking in hot water. Adding salt to the water can alleviate this.

• Baths dehydrate the body, and if you drink alcohol before or during a bath you'll get even more dehydrated. Replenish the fluid you've lost by drinking a few glasses of water after bathing.

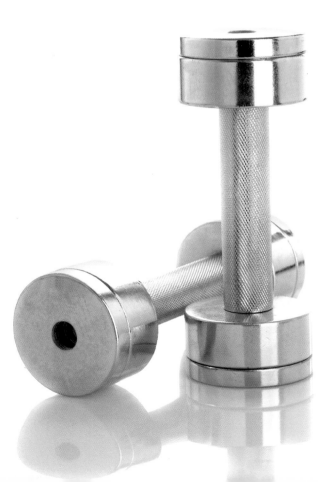

HEALING WITH EXERCISE: MOVEMENT THERAPY

Be active! It's no secret that exercise is a vital component of overall well-being. Don't fret about the sedentary life you may have been leading; now is always a good time to start increasing your physical activity.

While regular exercise is widely known as an effective way to control weight and tone muscles, medical studies have shown it provides many other benefits, including:

• Increases energy
• Stimulates the metabolism
• Oxygenates all the organs
• Helps digestion
• Decreases anxiety, tension, and depression
• Aids in the elimination of toxins and wastes
• Elevates levels of HDL, the "good" cholesterol
• Strengthens the heart, lungs, bones, muscles, and cartilage
• Improves circulation, mental clarity, and quality of sleep
• Keeps joints moving, which reduces chronic back pain and arthritic discomfort
• Releases endorphins, neurotransmitters that lower blood pressure, generate a sense of euphoria, and serve as a strong analgesic

Before embarking on any exercise program, consult your physician and undergo a thorough physical exam. You don't want to engage in movements or levels of activity that may cause a problem or aggravate an

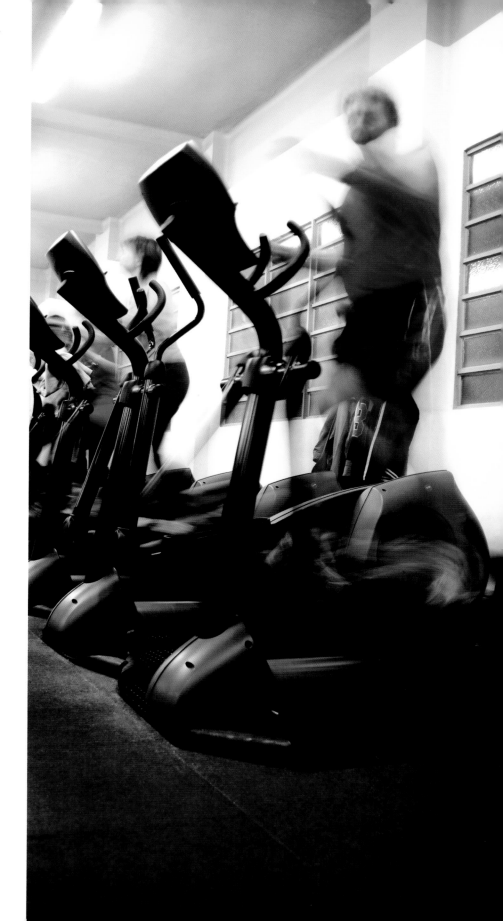

RIGHT: Your health plan should include some kind of aerobic exercise for a minimum of thirty minutes three to five times a week.

existing one. You'll likely be more successful if you find a pastime you enjoy. There are dozens of options, including swimming, jogging, hiking, biking, bowling, dancing, tennis, soccer, horseback riding, martial arts, racquetball, basketball, and volleyball.

To achieve results, you need to exercise a minimum of thirty minutes three to five times a week. Plan on five minutes to warm up, five minutes to reach your target heart rate, at least fifteen minutes to maintain activity at that rate, and five minutes to cool down. Start slow and set realistic goals; it'll take a few weeks for you to build up to your desired regimen.

Exercise energizes, so avoid doing it right before you retire or you probably will have a difficult time sleeping. Other than that, any time is a good time to exercise. Consistency is key; it's best to set aside the same time every day so it becomes an established routine. If for some reason you can't exercise at that hour on a particular day, don't skip it. Find another open slot to do it and go back to your normal schedule the next day.

If you absolutely can't squeeze in a formal session, be as active as possible that day. Climb stairs rather than take the elevator. Park your car as far as you can from your destination and walk the rest of the way. Pick up litter, rake your yard, or vacuum your house.

Instead of viewing exercise as a chore, make it fun. Do it to music. Vary your regimen so you don't get bored. Make it a social event; exercise with friends, family members, business associates, or a group with similar interests and goals so you have the support you need to keep motivated.

twelve extraordinary indulgences

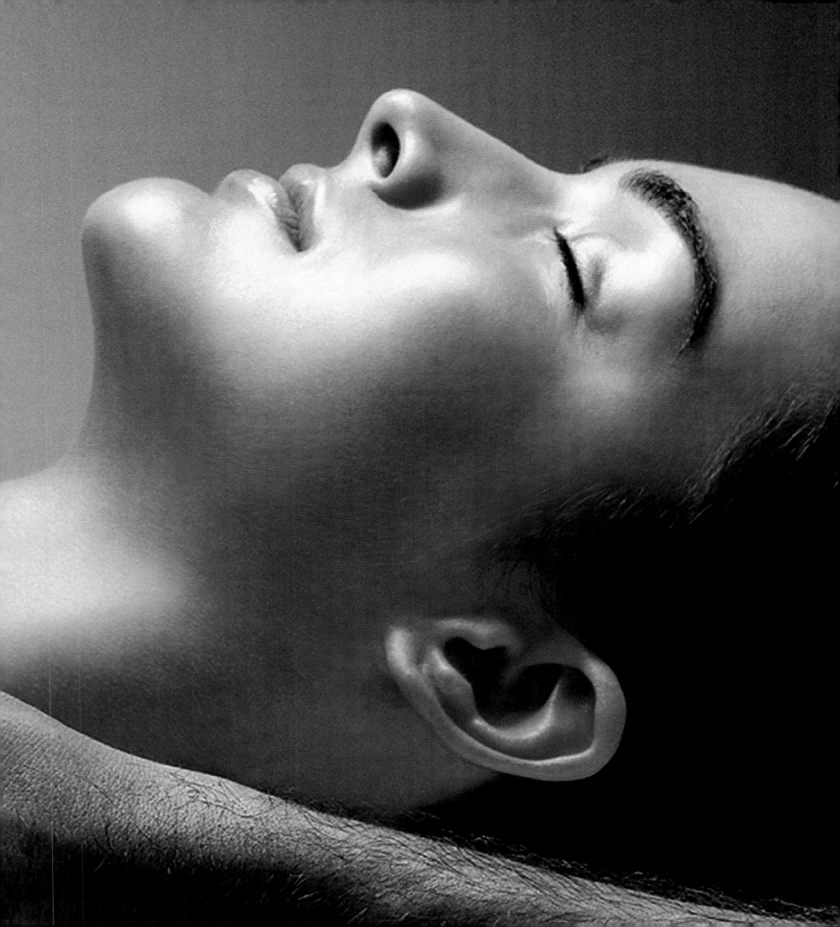

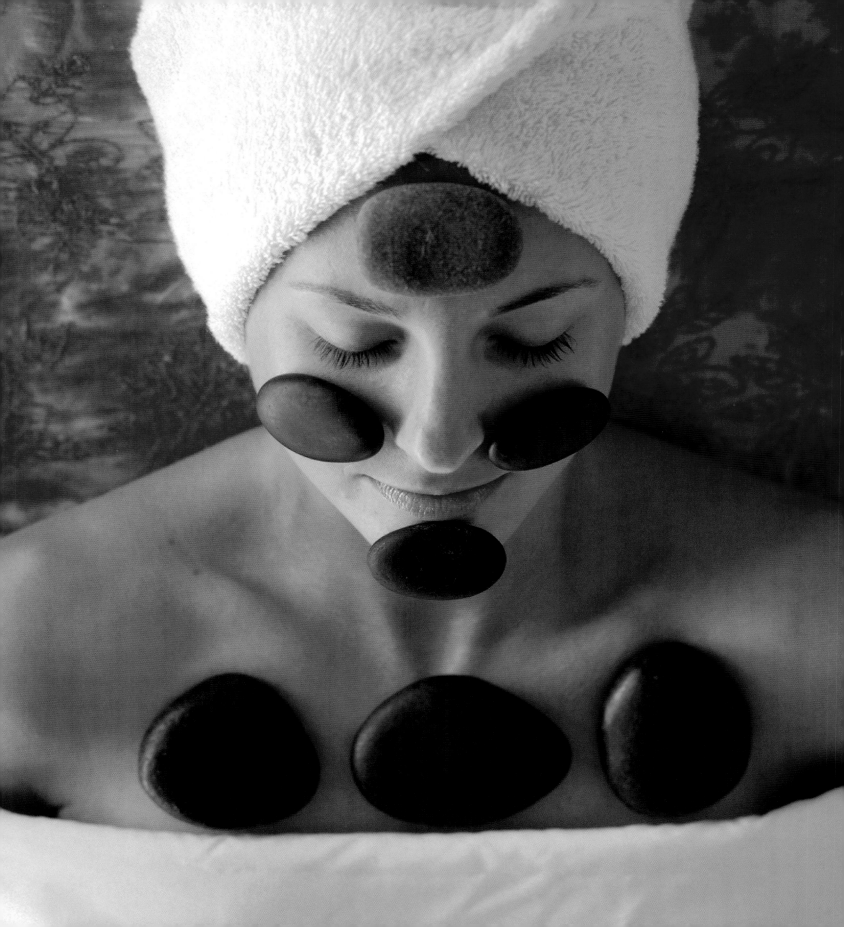

c h a p t e r   6

The healing begins the moment you step into a spa's welcoming embrace. Heavenly fragrances—ylang-ylang, neroli, bergamot and more—waft through the air with the gentle voices of the flute, piano, guitar, and violin. Bowls of fresh fruits and vases of flowers adorn tables and countertops. Lounges open to the ocean or gardens of vivid greenery.

Your pace slows along with your pulse. Gone are thoughts of bills, meetings, errands, and deadlines. You've begun to succumb to the serenity of the spa.

From massages, facials, and baths to masks, wraps, and exfoliations, spa menus have been designed to relax and rejuvenate. Unique ingredients, settings, implements, or techniques set the following twelve treatments apart from the hundreds offered at fine facilities throughout Hawai'i.

PRECEDING SPREAD: You'll "float" face up on two water pillows for the entire fifty-minute Hydrotherm Massage at Aveda Lifestyle Salon & Spa.

LEFT: A private after-hours session at The Spa at Four Seasons Resort Lāna'i at Mānele Bay includes your choice of six treatments, including the Stone Facial.

AFTER-HOURS PAMPERING

The only way a first-class spa experience could be better is if you have the whole fabulous facility to yourself. The Spa After Hours Experience comes close by offering a private two-hour session for between two and eight guests.

Two days' notice is required. On the day of your appointment, the spa will close at its regular time of 7:00 p.m. so the staff can make preparations for your party's exclusive visit. When the spa reopens at 7:30 p.m., an attendant will greet you with pineapple tea.

Sip your tea while a therapist massages your neck and shoulders. This is followed by a fifty-minute treatment

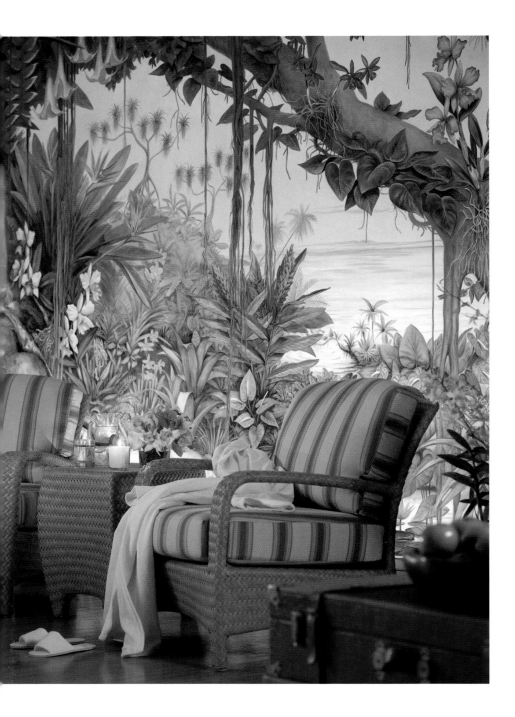

of your choice; options include Banana Coconut Scrub, Pineapple Citrus Polish, Limu (Seaweed) Body Mask, Ti Leaf Wrap, Hot Stone Massage, and Stone Facial.

Then relax in the eucalyptus steam room and red cedar sauna before showering and concluding your experience with light appetizers. The menu usually includes a green salad, Asian chicken skewers, papaya fruit bowl, and pineapple and shrimp kebobs, but it can be altered to accommodate your special dietary needs.

The Spa
Four Seasons Resort Lāna'i at Mānele Bay
One Mānele Bay Road
Lāna'i City, Lāna'i
(808) 565-2000
www.fourseasons.com/manelebay

LEFT: Vivid handpainted murals depicting orchids, anthuriums, heliconias, and other tropical flora decorate The Spa's lounge.

FOR CHOCOLATE LOVERS

Here's a way couples can savor a whole pot of chocolate without gaining an ounce. Exploration in Chocolate is a decadent two-and-a-half-hour indulgence for two that begins with a side-by-side massage in a deluxe spa suite (you'll each have your own therapist).

After the massage, the therapists apply a body scrub made of sugar, macadamia nuts, macadamia nut oil, and unsweetened dark chocolate that's good enough to eat. You'll then be left alone for over an hour as you awaken your playful selves with the remaining chocolate macadamia nut scrub. Listen to music, soak in the private Jacuzzi tub on the *lānai* (veranda), sip tea—it's the ultimate quiet time *à deux*.

This treatment takes you and your sweetheart on a memorable journey away from your hectic everyday lives. It is aromatic, it exfoliates the skin, it detoxifies and promotes new cell growth, and, of course, it is very romantic.

Mandara Spa
Hilton Hawaiian Village Beach Resort & Spa
2005 Kālia Road
Waikīkī, O'ahu
(808) 945-7721
www.mandaraspa.com

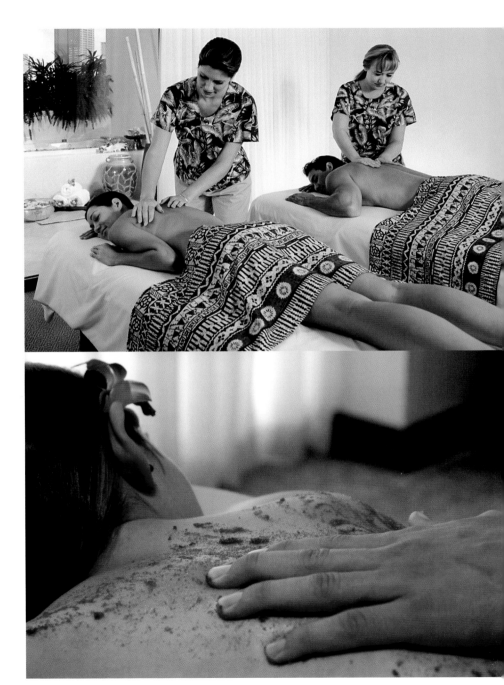

TOP RIGHT: Couples' heavenly Exploration in Chocolate begins with a side-by-side massage.

BOTTOM RIGHT: They're then left alone for over an hour to discover the sensuous delights of chocolate.

BELOW: Set aside at least seven consecutive days for Pancha Karma pampering, which includes synchronized massages by two therapists.

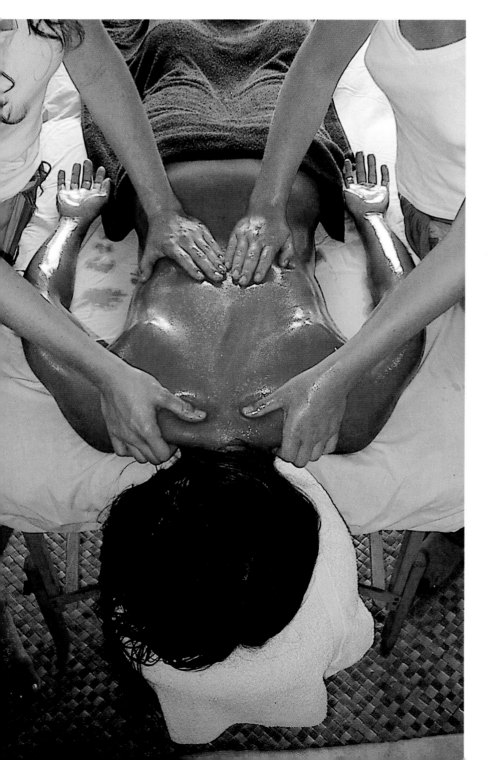

GOOD KARMA

Got a week of free time? If so, consider the cleansing rejuvenation program called Pancha Karma, which is the cornerstone of Ayurveda. A healing tradition that originated in India more than five thousand years ago, Ayurveda is based on the premise that to be healthy you must achieve harmony in all aspects of your life.

To gain the most from Pancha Karma, at least seven consecutive days of treatments are recommended (the program can be extended to twenty-one consecutive days). By experiencing two to three hours of such attention daily, you'll gradually move into a complete state of balance in body, mind, and spirit.

Every day, you'll receive a synchronized warm oil massage by two therapists followed by a full-body steam bath and your choice of other treatments such as herbal rubs, detoxification body wraps, and *shirodhara*, during which a stream of warm herbal oil is gently poured on your forehead.

Ayurveda and yoga enthusiasts believe there are seven chakras (energy centers) in the body. The forehead supposedly is the entrance to the sixth chakra, the "third eye" associated with wisdom and spiritual insight. Warm oil poured on this point transports you to a deep state of relaxation, removes stress, steadies your emotions, and sharpens your senses. It also alleviates insomnia, headaches, depression, panic attacks, and addictions. You'll emerge feeling as though you've just completed a long, blissful meditation session.

Ayurveda Center of Hawai'i
Hanalei Colony Resort
5-7132 Kūhiō Highway
Hā'ena, Kaua'i
(808) 826-6621
www.panchakarma.net

BELOW (FROM LEFT):
Rose quartz, snowflake
obsidian, and rock
crystal combs stimulate
chakras and meridians
on the head to achieve
health benefits.

TENDING YOUR HAIR GARDEN

Throughout the world, throughout the ages, humans have adorned their bodies, homes, and places of worship with gemstones and crystals, which are treasured both for their beauty and for their ability to heal. Holistic practitioners believe when these semiprecious minerals come in contact with the chakras and acupuncture meridians that run across the head and body, total well-being can be attained.

Think of the hair as a garden and the scalp as the "earth" in which "hair plants" grow. When we gently cleanse, nourish, and stimulate the hair and scalp with products made from pure, natural ingredients, the hair blossoms—and so do we.

The simple act of combing your hair with gemstone combs supposedly can uplift, balance, and energize your body. For example, rose quartz is said to dissipate anger, resentment, jealousy, and fear and turn them into self-confidence and love. In addition, it addresses concerns related to the heart, kidneys, circulatory system, fertility, migraines, and sexual dysfunction.

Rock crystal is said to enhance mental capacity, clarity, and concentration. In holistic medicine, it often is used to treat dizziness, headaches, and digestive problems.

Use the snowflake obsidian comb to remove negative feelings and thoughts. It also has been used to alleviate pain resulting from arthritis and scar tissue.

In China, jade has long been a symbol of strength, wisdom, peace, and harmony. It has a centering and calming effect, and purportedly is beneficial to the heart, the flow and quality of blood, and kidney and bladder function (thus preventing the formation of stones).

Hair Garden
P.O. Box 1032
Kula, Maui
(808) 250-9115
www.hairgarden.com

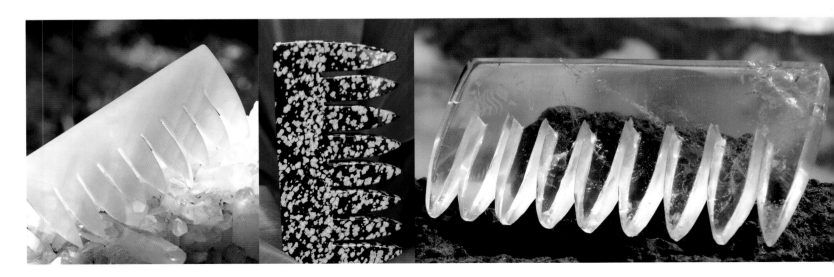

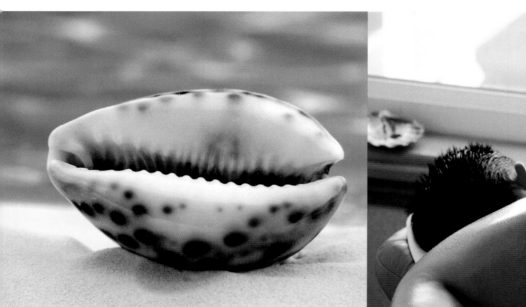

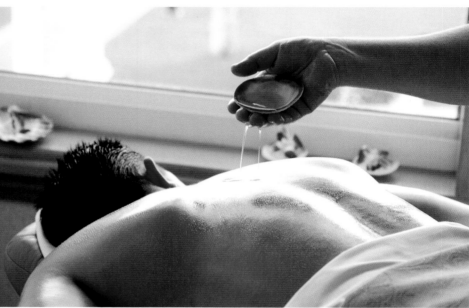

INCREDIBLE SHELLWORK

Seashells were the ancient Hawaiians' jewels. Women scoured beaches for the prettiest specimens, and strung them into necklaces and bracelets using a fine cord of *olonā* (a native shrub). Long ago, shells also were made into utilitarian items such as fishhooks, lures, food scrapers, and trumpets for communication (the sound of a conch could carry as far as two miles).

Modern-day healing practitioners at Spa Grande go one step further, employing cowrie, abalone, conch, and *'opihi* (limpet) shells of various sizes, shapes, and textures in an innovative fifty- or eighty-minute Seashell Massage. Through a cupping process, the therapist first uses heated seashells to warm your body, promote deep relaxation, and stimulate the flow of energy (the shells are filled with a volcanic compound that keeps them warm up to one hour).

Following this, she applies rich *kukui* nut, macadamia nut, and coconut oils, then massages your skin with a combination of shells, using long, rhythmic strokes. She fits small, textured shells in between your toes and fingers, and glides smooth larger ones across your back, legs, and arms.

Therapists select their own shells, and although they may have the same types of shells in their personal collections, no two are exactly alike—thus, no Seashell Massage is ever exactly alike.

Spa Grande

Grand Wailea Resort Hotel & Spa
3850 Alanui Drive
Wailea, Maui
(808) 875-1234
www.grandwailea.com

BELOW: The gentle rocking motion you feel as you rest on two warm water pillows adds to the pleasure of the Hydrotherm Massage.

PILLOW TALK

Imagine a table topped with two large water pillows heated to about 104 degrees. Then imagine yourself floating face up on top of this undulating water bed as a massage therapist coaxes the kinks out of your body.

Unlike other treatments where you're asked to turn so the therapist can reach different parts of your body, you'll stay in this position throughout the entire fifty-minute Hydrotherm Massage. The warmth envelops you like a blanket as the therapist kneads, hits pressure points, and uses long, flowing strokes to release impurities and tension in your muscles and tissues. She also may use dragging and circular motions and "scoop" beneath you, using your weight to assist with pressure.

The subtle movement of the water pillows adds to the pleasure of the experience. It's like you're being gently rocked—like you're floating on your back in the ocean and the water is lapping around you. The constant heat is nurturing; you feel tranquil, comforted, safe, and very, very relaxed.

Aveda Lifestyle Salon & Spa
Ala Moana Center
1450 Ala Moana Boulevard
Honolulu, O'ahu
(808) 947-6141
www.aveda.com

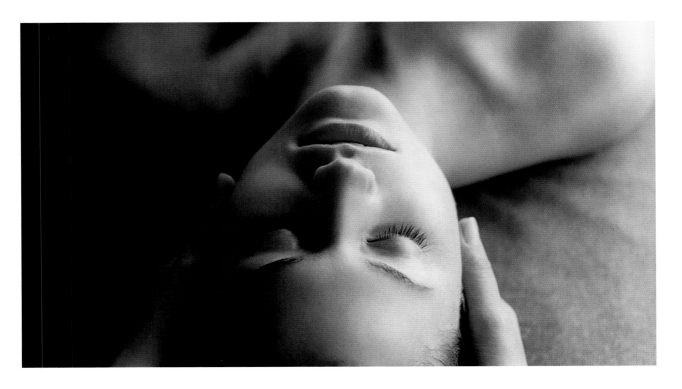

COLOR YOUR WORLD

Red to energize, blue to calm, green to soothe aching muscles, orange to promote happiness—instead of downing pills to achieve well-being, try a prescription of color.

The therapeutic power of colors has been known around the world for centuries. Each shade of the spectrum—violet, indigo, blue, green, yellow, orange, and red—supposedly has its own specific "frequency" that corresponds to one of the body's seven chakras that govern our physical condition and state of mind.

For the twenty-five-minute Deluxe Thalassotherapy with Color and Essential Oils, color light therapy is combined with thalassotherapy, which uses ocean water pumped directly from nearby lagoons. As you recline in a thalasso tub, you're massaged with a series of adjustable underwater hydro and air jets that automatically cycle through six different areas of your body, from shoulders to feet. The jet action improves circulation, and the seawater softens, remineralizes, and nourishes the skin. Seawater contains several of the same trace minerals that are found in human plasma, including oxygen, hydrogen, and iodine.

Throughout the treatment, underwater beams of color are directed at you. Depending on the results desired, one color may be used the whole time or different colors may be rotated. Aromatherapy oils boost the healing effects of the color rays; choose from detoxification, serenity, vital energy, and antistress oils.

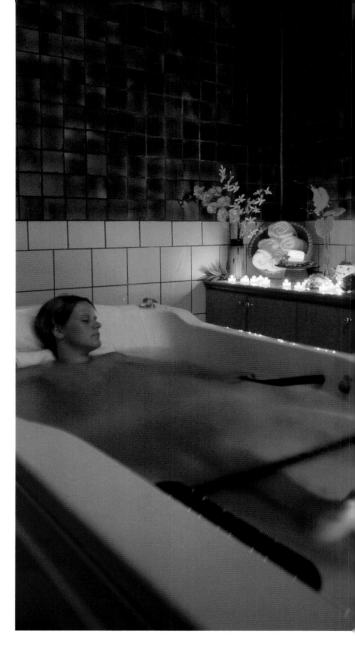

Ihilani Spa
JW Marriott Ihilani Resort & Spa
92-1001 Olani Street
Kapolei, O'ahu
(808) 679-3321
www.ihilani.com

ABOVE: The Deluxe Thalassotherapy combines the therapeutic powers of colors and an underwater massage from jets of air and seawater.

BELOW: Lava Watsu incorporates acupressure, stretching, and massage in a solar-heated pool.

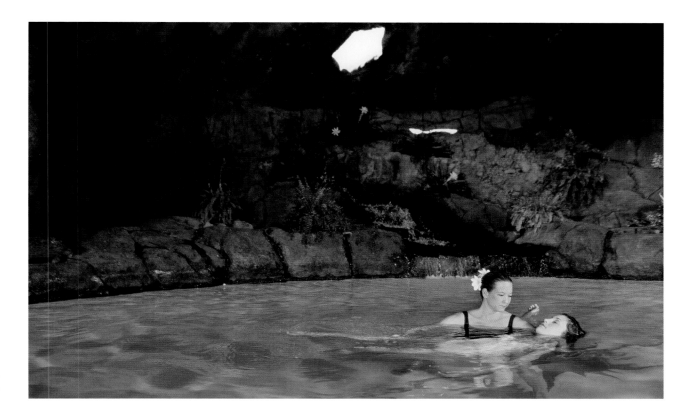

WATER MAGIC

Kahi Kīkaha means "place of soaring," and that's exactly the sensation you'll get during aquatic body therapy in this one-thousand-square-foot solar-heated pool. Nestled in a garden of Hawaiian medicinal plants among natural lava tubes—the wombs of the *'āina* (land), according to ancient belief—it is the only pool of its kind in the state.

For the fifty- or eighty-minute Lava Watsu treatment, you'll float on your back as your therapist leads you in a slow, graceful dance around the pool, stopping on occasion to press key acupressure points; to lift and stretch your back; and to massage your hands, arms, legs, and feet. Each well-choreographed sequence in the body-temperature salt water is accompanied by soothing underwater acoustics and lighting effects.

As your trust in the therapist and the process grows, so does your level of relaxation. Releasing control, living only in the moment, being liberated from stress and pain—that is the gift of this water work. More and more tension in your body melts away until you feel as free and flowing as the water itself.

Mauna Lani Spa
Mauna Lani Resort
68-1365 Pauoa Road
Kohala Coast, Big Island
(808) 881-7922
www.maunalani.com

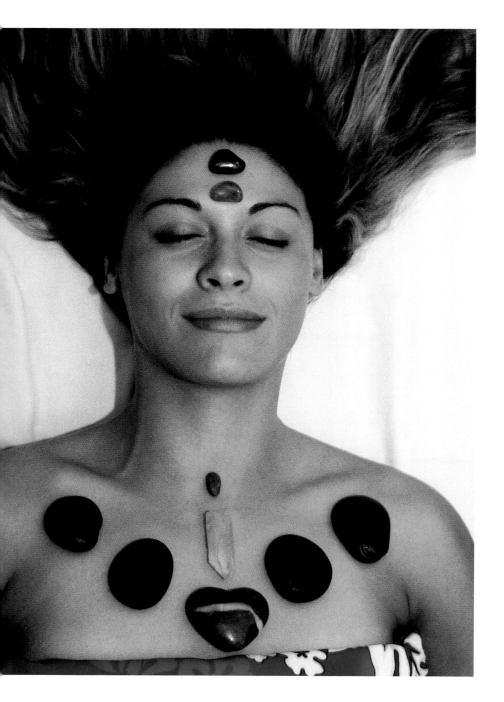

A JEWEL OF A TREATMENT

Quartz, turquoise, amethyst, hematite—the Eurostone Anti-Stress Aromatherapy Facial stimulates your lymphatic system and balances your energy centers with select gemstones and heated and chilled river stones. They're placed on key acupressure points on your face and upper chest to release healing energies.

Used in conjunction with a blend of pure essential oils and botanicals, the smaller stones are ideal for small spaces, such as around the eyes, while the larger ones are used to massage facial tissue. As the rocks and stones are gently manipulated on your face, minerals are drawn out and absorbed by the skin. The result is an overall sense of restful relaxation.

The basic philosophy behind this fifty-minute facial is that the body is composed of two opposite energies—yin and yang. It is believed that the health of the skin, mind, and body can be optimally achieved when these energies are in balance with each other. Relaxation, emotional release, mental clarity, and a radiant complexion are among the benefits of this effective holistic treatment.

Waikīkī Plantation Spa
Outrigger Waikīkī on the Beach
2335 Kalākaua Avenue
Waikīkī, Oʻahu
(808) 926-2880
www.outrigger.com

BELOW LEFT: During the Kaua'i Clay Ritual, a mask of Kaua'i clay, *'awa*, organic aloe, and *noni* purifies and moisturizes the skin.

BELOW RIGHT: That's followed by a rinse in an outdoor lava rock shower and a relaxing full-body massage.

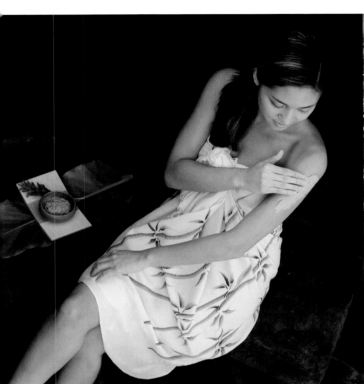
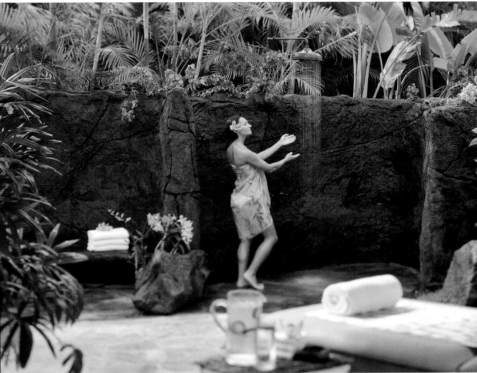

HEAVEN ON EARTH

There's something heavenly about making a connection with the earth, and the 110-minute Kaua'i Clay Ritual enables you to do that. To start, warm coconut oil is drizzled over your body as you lie in an open-air, thatched-roof teak *hale* (bungalow). *'Awa* (kava) is then lightly sprinkled and rubbed in with hot stones to exfoliate and smooth your skin.

Next, a mask of mineral-rich Kaua'i clay infused with *'awa*, organic aloe, and *noni* (Indian mulberry) is applied. As your body is wrapped in warm towels to seal in the purifying and moisturizing ingredients, relax and quiet your mind as you listen to the music of chirping birds, rustling leaves, and a cascading waterfall.

After rinsing in an outdoor lava rock shower (carefully situated to allow complete privacy, of course), you'll enjoy a full-body massage that coaxes all the kinks from your muscles and joints, and drenches your skin with a wonderful cream scented with tropical botanicals.

Anara Spa
Grand Hyatt Kaua'i Resort & Spa
1571 Po'ipū Road
Po'ipū, Kaua'i
(808) 240-6440
www.anaraspa.com

BELOW (FROM LEFT): The heat from *ganban-yoku* releases toxins from the body, making it a wonderful prelude to a massage. After your *ganban-yoku* and massage treatments, enjoy a fragrant Coconut Lemongrass Bath Soak.

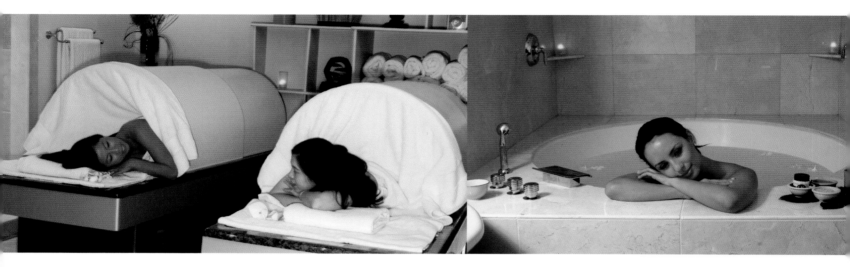

STONE BATH

Technically, *ganban-yoku* (stone bath) is not a bath because it doesn't involve water. Even so, the benefits from this treatment, which originated in Japan, are identical: It cleanses the body, increases blood circulation, and stimulates the production of collagen, leaving the skin smooth and shiny. Proponents of *ganban-yoku* also believe it activates the metabolism; burns calories, making it useful for weight control; and relieves stiff shoulders, back and joint pain, and other circulatory problems.

For the Glow and Refresh *ganban-yoku* treatment, you'll wear light, loose clothing and lie on an Indian granite table warmed to 103 degrees (unlike the intense heat of a sauna, the safe far-infrared rays that emanate from the stone are quite relaxing). Within thirty minutes, as the heat penetrates deep into your body, you'll experience a profuse sweat that flushes out toxins. At the same time, you'll reap the benefits of the table's herbal steam dome, which covers your body up to your shoulders.

Although "infrared" may sound intimidating, there's no cause for concern; it's simply a form of invisible energy that transmits heat from one object to another without a liquid or solid conductor. The sun is our principal source of infrared heat.

Those who've tried *ganban-yoku* like it because they work up a good sweat without exercising or enduring extreme heat. Even better, unlike the sweat produced when you lounge in a sauna or engage in prolonged physical activity, the sweat from *ganban-yoku* supposedly isn't sticky so you don't need to shower afterward. Glow and Refresh is marvelous on its own or as a prelude to a deep-tissue massage.

Spa Pure
The Wyland Waikīkī
400 Royal Hawaiian Avenue
Waikīkī, Oʻahu
(808) 924-3200
www.spapurewaikiki.com

A HEALING DANCE

The early Hawaiians had no concept of disease; to them, illness indicated the afflicted person was out of alignment with *hā* (breath of life) and the rhythm of nature. Balance those, they believed, and good health was ensured. Techniques to realign *hā* were passed down from generation to generation, some of which are employed in the 110-minute Hawaiian Ceremonial Lomilomi.

As in days of old, this memorable massage is based on *aloha lōkahi* (love and unity), which essentially means living in harmony with yourself, others, and nature. Every thought, every action, should reflect respect and appreciation for all things, both animate and inanimate.

The treatment is performed in an open-air, thatched-roof *hale* set beside the sea. At least two practitioners (up to four can be arranged) apply a liberal amount of oil on your body with their hands and forearms, using strokes that range from light and fast to slow and deep. One element of this synchronized bodywork emulates the graceful flight of the *'iwa* (frigate bird), which is known for its ability to soar to great heights and for long distances without landing.

Skilled partners in healing, the therapists choreograph their movements to ancient chants and traditional and contemporary Hawaiian music. The results of their efforts: peace, enhanced awareness, and unrestrained pleasure and joy.

The Spa at Four Seasons Resort Maui
Four Seasons Resort Maui at Wailea
3900 Wailea Alanui
Wailea, Maui
(808) 874-2925
www.fourseasons.com/maui

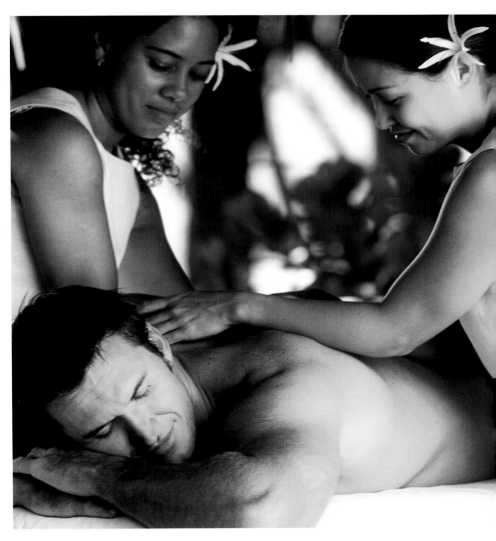

ABOVE: In an open-air thatched-roof *hale* beside the sea, two massage therapists choreograph their movements to the sounds of ancient chants and traditional and contemporary Hawaiian music.

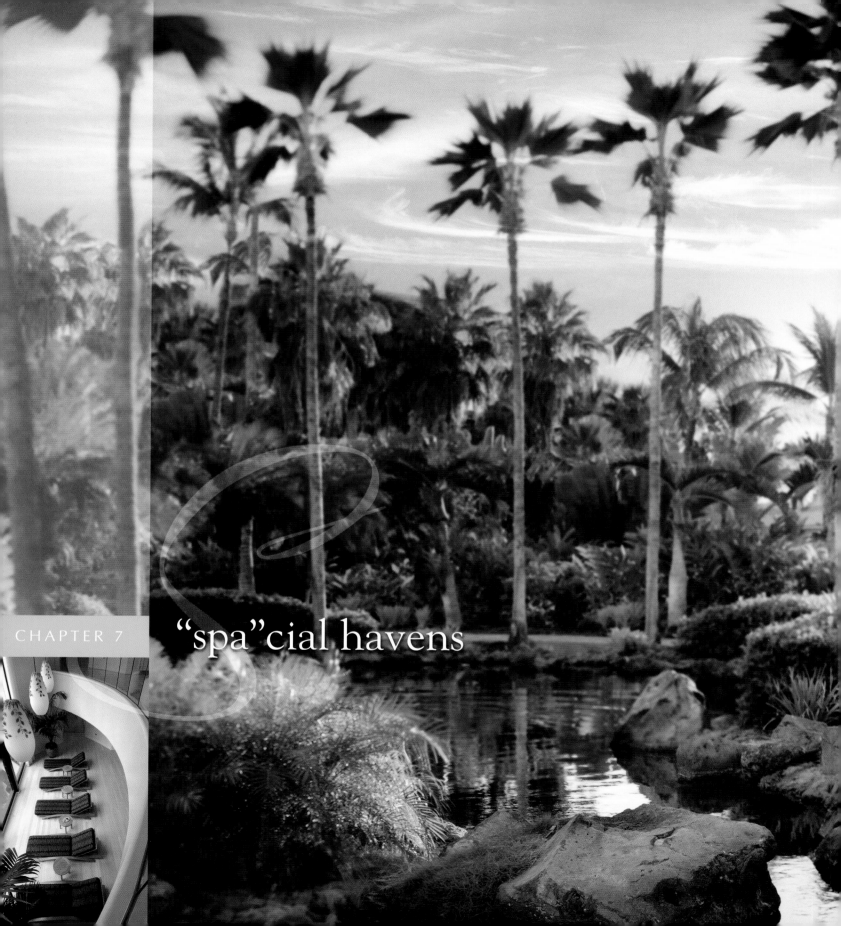

"spa"cial havens

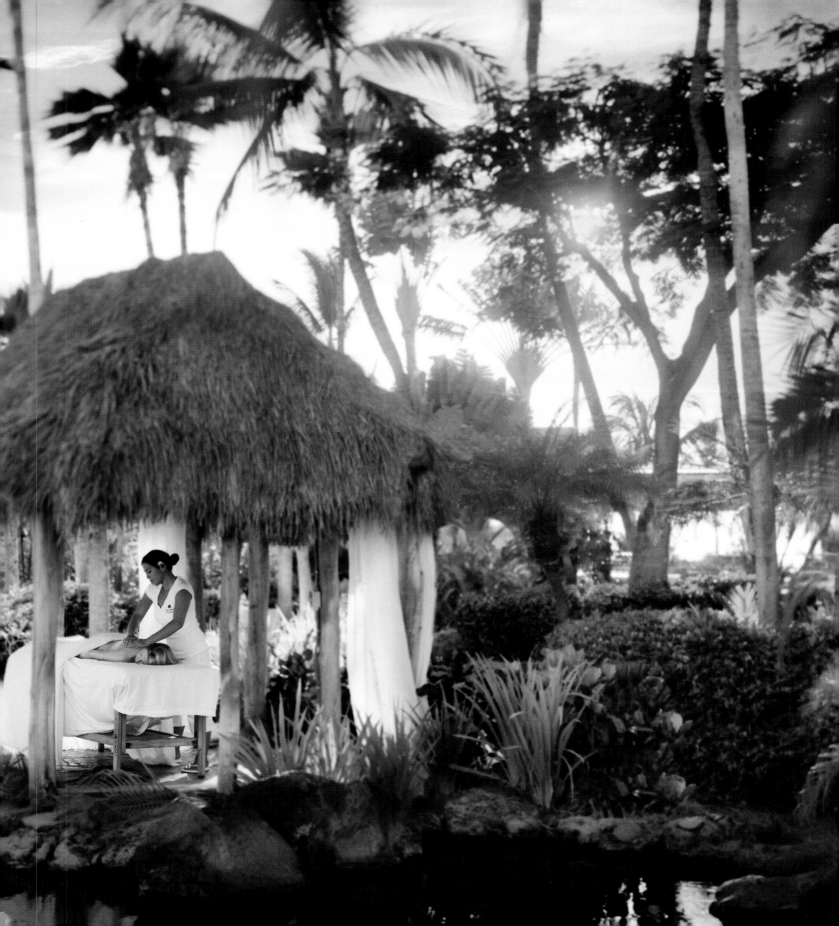

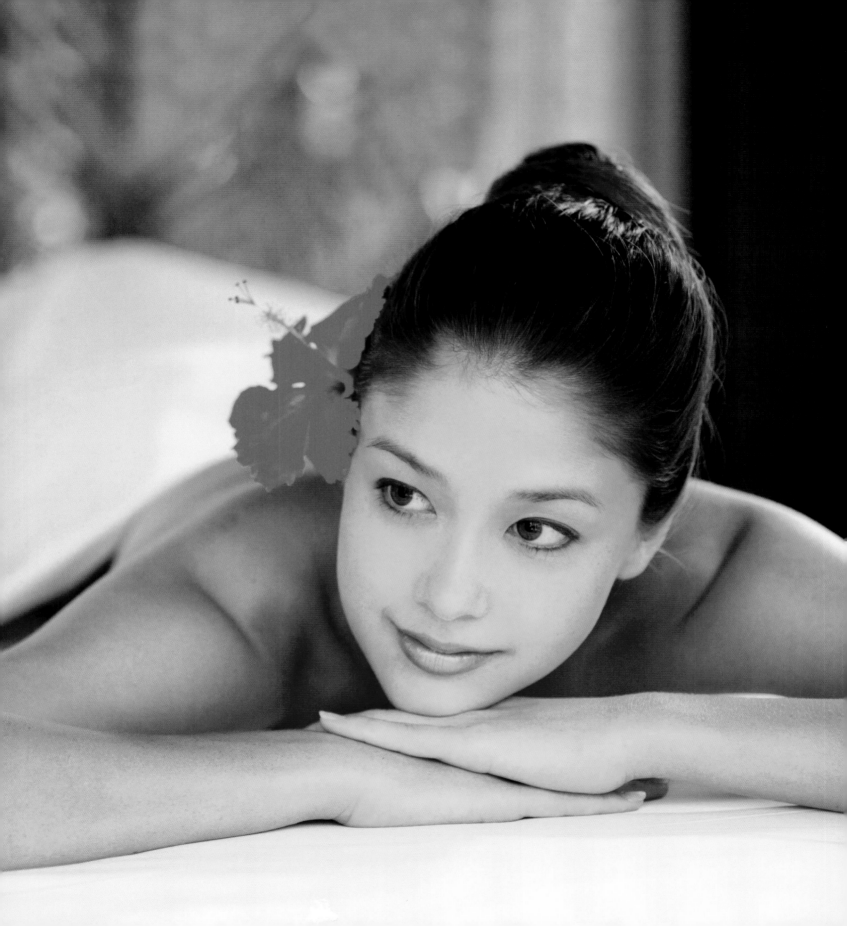

chapter 7

Following is a comprehensive roundup of spa facilities in Hawai'i. Some are grand in size with luxurious appointments. Others are intimate and modest. All promise a relaxing escape from the cares of everyday life.

O'ahu

abhasa

The Royal Hawaiian
2259 Kalākaua Avenue
Honolulu, Hawai'i 96815
(808) 922-8200
www.abhasa.com

Facility highlights: Eleven treatment areas, including three couples' cabanas in the garden; relaxation patio in the garden; two steam rooms; Jacuzzi; full-service hair, nail, and makeup salon

Special services: Body wraps in cocoon beds (akin to water beds); specialized facials for wrinkles, pigmentation, acne, scars, and rosacea

Signature treatment: Lomilomi Garden Massage

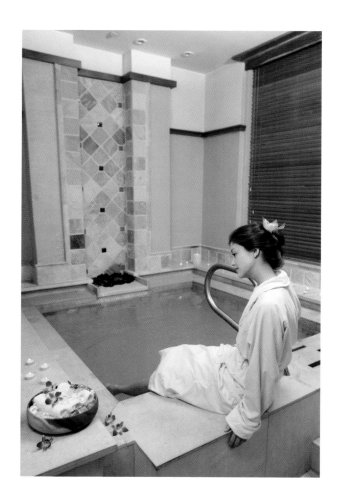

PRECEDING SPREAD: At Spa Grande, you can enjoy a massage outdoors in a lush, tropical setting. INSET: Lounge chairs at Nā Ho'olā Spa face the ocean.

LEFT: It's easy to relax in the oasis of peace and beauty that is abhasa.

RIGHT: abhasa's Jacuzzi is a great place to linger either before or after your treatment.

Ampy's: A Day Spa

1441 Kapi'olani Boulevard, Suite 377
Honolulu, Hawai'i 96814
(808) 946-3838
www.ampys.com

Facility highlights: Fifteen treatment rooms, including one for couples; dry sauna; manicure/pedicure station; relaxation room; aesthetic school for vocational training

Special services: Teen services, organic facials, ultrasonic microdermabrasion, cold laser treatment

Signature treatment: Maui Mango and Alpha Hydroxy Body Polish

Aveda Lifestyle Salon & Spa

Ala Moana Center
1450 Ala Moana Boulevard
Honolulu, Hawai'i 96814
(808) 947-6141
www.aveda.com

Facility highlights: Six treatment rooms, including one wet room with Vichy shower; full-service salon; separate nail salon; relaxation areas for men and women; men's and women's eucalyptus steam rooms

Special services: All spa services come with a footbath and foot massage with your choice of essential oil. All salon services come with a hand/arm massage and moisturizing treatment; a stress-relief treatment on the head, neck, and shoulders; and use of an aroma-infused towel for men and a makeup touch-up for women. All salon, spa, and retail guests are offered Aveda Comforting Tea and may request a complimentary stress-relief massage on the massage chair in the retail area (no purchase is necessary). Day packages include lunch catered by Neiman Marcus.

Signature treatment: Aveda Hydrotherm Massage

Elements Spa & Salon

1726 Kapi'olani Boulevard, Suite 206
Honolulu, Hawai'i 96814
(808) 942-0033
www.elementshawaii.com

Facility highlights: Three treatment rooms, including one for couples; full-service beauty salon

Special services: All services include complimentary extras; for example, haircuts include a mini facial and a scalp, neck, head, and shoulder massage, and one-hour facials include a complimentary foot treatment. There are seasonal specials and customized packages, and the spa can be reserved for showers, corporate events, and private parties.

Signature treatment: Sircuit Skin Signature Facial

Hawaiian Rainforest Salon & Spa

Pacific Beach Hotel
2490 Kalākaua Avenue
Honolulu, Hawai'i 96815
(808) 441-4890
www.hawaiianrainforest.com

Facility highlights: Four treatment rooms, including one for couples and a wet room with Vichy shower; sauna; steam room; full-service salon

Special services: All spa services begin with Aroma Bliss, an aromatherapy experience using your choice of essential oil.

Signature treatment: Nature's Wonder Green Tea Total Beauty

Heaven on Earth Salon & Day Spa

1050 Alakea Street
Honolulu, Hawai'i 96813
(808) 599-5501
www.heavenonearthhawaii.com

Facility highlights: Twelve treatment rooms, including one for couples and a Vichy wet treatment room; three pedicure/manicure stations; full-service salon; lounge areas to accommodate small groups or parties

Special services: Full-service makeup bar; permanent makeup; eyelash and hair extensions; eyelash perming; acupuncture; chemical peels; Botox treatments; microdermabrasion; corporate spa programs; portable massage chair for in-office visits in downtown Honolulu; *pau hana* (after work) amenities, including complimentary champagne with pedicures and complimentary wine with other services

Signature treatment: Lomilomi Massage

Ihilani Spa

JW Marriott Ihilani Resort & Spa
92-1001 Olani Street
Kapolei, Hawai'i 96707
(808) 679-3321
www.ihilani.com

Facility highlights: Nineteen treatment rooms, full-service salon and fitness center, outdoor lap pool, six championship tennis courts, two relaxation lounges, steam rooms, saunas, needle shower pavilions, Roman pools

Special services: Spa cuisine menu served in the relaxation lounges; Hip on *Hula*, one-on-one personal training incorporating basic *hula* movements; holistic Neuro Spa Program, which combines kinesiology, nutritional analysis, chiropractic, neuroemotional techniques, and

more; Ihilani Teens Club, designed to educate preteens and teens, aged eleven through eighteen, about health and wellness in a fun atmosphere. Options include Dueling Blenders, which show them how to create delicious smoothies.

Signature treatment: Deluxe Thalassotherapy with Color and Essential Oils

Lomilomi Hana Lima Healing Center and Spa

315 Uluniu Street, Suite 202
Kailua, Hawai'i 96734
(808) 263-0303
www.lomilomihanalima.com, www.lomilomialoha.com

Facility highlights: Four treatment rooms; relaxation room; private steam bath; private air bathtub for Hawaiian salt, aromatherapy, and color therapy treatments (its small air jets create relaxing water movement similar to a Jacuzzi)

Special services: Organic facials, complimentary tea service, custom essential oil blends, spa packages and parties, mother/child spa days, *ho'oponopono* sessions and other educational classes, Color and Aromatherapy Hydro Bath Experience with air jets and healing colors, Hawaiian salt, and essential oil

Signature treatment: Lomilomi Ola

Mandara Spa

Hilton Hawaiian Village Beach Resort & Spa
2005 Kālia Road
Honolulu, Hawai'i 96815
(808) 945-7721
www.mandaraspa.com

Facility highlights: Twenty-five treatment rooms, including one triple suite and five for couples; two Vichy showers; Hawaiian- and Balinese-themed furniture, decor, menu items, and ingredients used in treatments

Special services: Children's salon services such as manicures, pedicures, and hairstyling (including cornrow braids with beads); YSPA Teen Program with massages, facials, scrubs, and more

Signature treatment: Exploration in Chocolate

Moana Lani Spa

Moana Surfrider, A Westin Resort
2365 Kalākaua Avenue
Honolulu, Hawaiʻi 96815
(808) 922-3111
www.moanalanispa.com

Facility highlights: The only oceanfront spa in Waikīkī, nine massage rooms, two couples' suites with private oceanfront *lānai* and whirlpool tubs, one body treatment room, one Vichy shower water therapy room, three facial rooms, twenty-four-hour fitness center

Special services: Every massage begins with the placement of a warm herbal pack on the neck and back to promote relaxation (the pack is filled with clove, lavender, rice, orange peel, and allspice)

Signature treatment: Kauaʻi Clay and Hawaiian Vanilla Ritual

Moku Ola Hawaiian Healing Center

Koko Marina Center
7192 Kalanianaʻole Highway, Suite D-201
Honolulu, Hawaiʻi 96825
(808) 394-6658
www.mokuolahawaii.com

Facility highlights: Four treatment rooms, including one for couples and one for seated *lomilomi* massages and foot scrubs—all overlooking the marina and Koʻolau mountains

Special services: Its mission is to share and perpetuate the Hawaiian culture through healing practices; for example, *lomilomi* treatments incorporate *lāʻau lapaʻau*. The center can be booked for informative gatherings about Hawaiian cultural practices as well as for strictly social events such as private parties.

Signature treatment: Lomi Ola

Nā Hoʻōla Spa

Hyatt Regency Waikīkī Resort & Spa
2424 Kalākaua Avenue
Honolulu, Hawaiʻi 96815
(808) 237-6330
www.waikiki.hyatt.com/hyatt/hotels/activities/spa

Facility highlights: Nineteen treatment rooms, twenty-four-hour fitness center, two-level relaxation area, saunas, views of Waikīkī Beach and the Koʻolau mountains

Special services: Hulacise, an aerobic workout incorporating basic *hula* steps

Signature treatment: Pōhaku Massage

Paul Brown's Spa Olakino*Salon

Waikīkī Beach Marriott Resort & Spa
2552 Kalākaua Avenue
Honolulu, Hawaiʻi 96815
(808) 924-2121
www.spaolakino.com

Facility highlights: Ten treatment rooms, one makeup station, three hairdressing stations, two manicure/pedicure stations, one couples' room with a Japanese *furo* tub, steam showers

Special services: Fresh pineapple and tea are served before every service

Signature treatment: Magic Island Massage

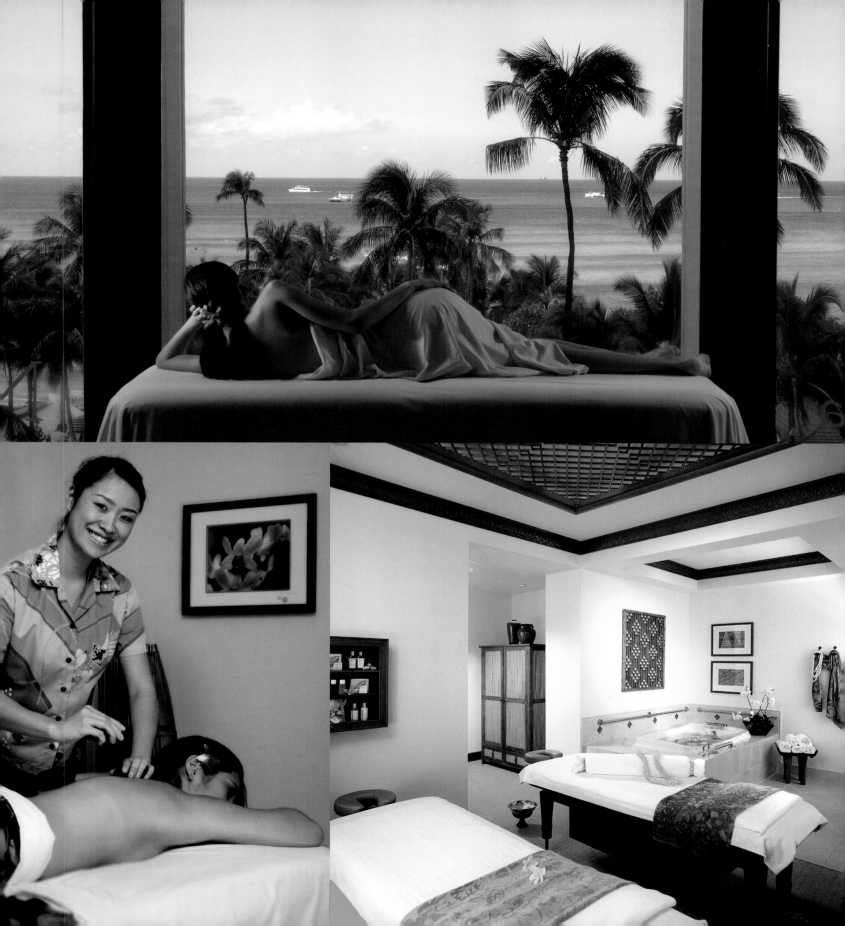

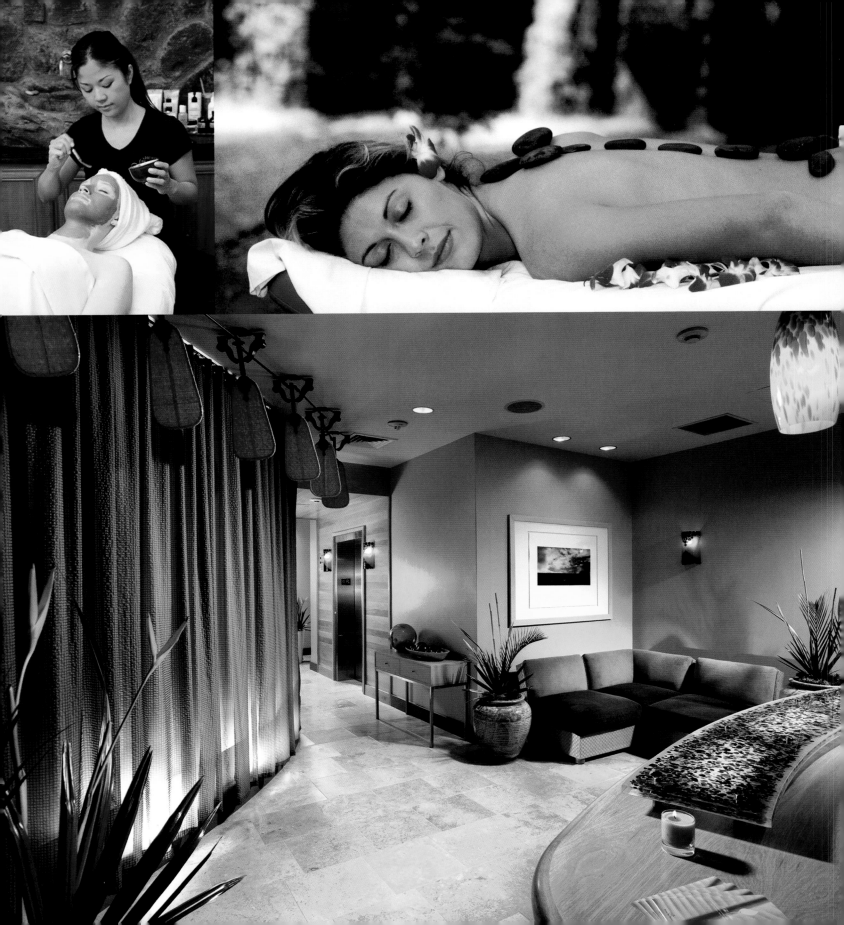

Serenity Spa Hawai'i

Outrigger Reef on the Beach
2169 Kālia Road
Honolulu, Hawai'i 96815
(808) 926-2882
www.serenityspahawaii.com

Facility highlights: Two-level spa has eight massage rooms, including two couples' suites with hydrotherapy tubs; three facial rooms; three hydrotherapy rooms; full-service salon; two relaxation lounges; men's and women's locker rooms with steam rooms

Special services: Private after-hour parties can be booked for birthdays, bridal showers, and girls' day out. The staff can create party favors and off-the-regular-menu services to fit your budget.

Signature treatment: Hot Shell Massage

Spa Luana

Turtle Bay Resort
57-091 Kamehameha Highway
Kahuku, Hawai'i 96731
(808) 447-6868
www.turtlebayresort.com

Facility highlights: One oceanfront cabana for couples' massages, six ocean-view treatment rooms, full-service salon, outdoor ocean-view yoga and relaxation areas, fitness center

Special services: Manicures and pedicures for children twelve years and younger

Signature treatment: Pineapple Pedicure

Spa Pure

The Wyland Waikīkī
400 Royal Hawaiian Avenue
Honolulu, Hawai'i 96815
(808) 924-3200
www.spapurewaikiki.com

Facility highlights: Three treatment rooms, including two for couples; one room with a soaking tub for therapeutic baths (it's large enough to accommodate two people); relaxation lanai; the only two *ganban-yoku* stone bath tables in Hawai'i (see details in chapter 6: Twelve Extraordinary Indulgences). All rooms are furnished with custom-made furniture, including curved maple mirror frames and onyx and marble back-splashes that reflect the spa's wave-inspired theme.

Special services: Massages beside a warm salt-water pool; in-room treatments; exclusive use of Phytoceane, a French line using Jania rubens, a red seaweed found off the coast of Brittany (France prohib-its shipping in the area to prevent the introduction of oil and other contaminants)

Signature treatment: Water to Land Combo Massage

Spa Suites

The Kāhala Hotel & Resort
5000 Kāhala Avenue
Honolulu, Hawai'i 96816
(808) 739-8938
www.kahalaresort.com

Facility highlights: Five private 550-square-foot Spa Suites (one for couples), each with a changing area, private shower, infinity-edged soaking bath, and private relaxation area with a courtyard landscaped with Ha-waiian flora

Special services: The Spa Suites concept provides you

with your own personal spa suite, offering the luxury of complete privacy; most treatments begin with a complimentary foot soak of *'alaea* salt and flower essences; teen spa parties, including a personal training session, massage, manicure, and pedicure

Signature treatment: Kala Ko'iko'i Lomilomi

SpaHalekūlani

Halekūlani Hotel
2199 Kālia Road
Honolulu, Hawai'i 96815
(808) 931-5322
www.halekulani.com

Facility highlights: Seven treatment rooms, including two suites for couples (one has a private shower and Japanese *furo* tub, the other has a garden terrace with a steam shower); full-service salon; retail boutique; ocean-view terrace relaxation area

Special services: Complimentary foot treatment and light refreshments with each spa experience; manicure and hair treatments use vegan and organic products; the teen spa menu offers makeup lessons, manicure/pedicure combinations, mini-facials, and applications of island-themed temporary tattoos; à la carte menu of fruit parfaits, salads, wraps, and other health-conscious options served on the terrace

Signature treatment: Polynesian Nonu

Waikīkī Plantation Spa

Outrigger Waikīkī on the Beach
2335 Kalākaua Avenue
Honolulu, Hawai'i 96815
(808) 926-2880
www.outrigger.com

Facility highlights: Bi-level rooftop locale includes six treatment rooms (two for couples), adjacent fitness center

Special services: Choose from seven ingredients for the Body Polish and Scrub treatment—macadamia nuts, pineapple, sugarcane, Kona coffee, Hawaiian salt, volcanic pumice, or green and white teas. All eight of their massage techniques can be booked as couples' treatments.

Signature treatment: Lomi Pōhaku Massage

Maui

Heavenly Spa by Westin

The Westin Kā'anapali Ocean Resort Villas
6 Kai Ala Drive
Kā'anapali, Hawai'i 96761
(808) 667-3200
www.westinkaanapali.com

Facility highlights: Thirteen treatment rooms, including three couples' massage suites and three hydrotherapy rooms; separate men's and women's lounges, each with a steam room; outdoor relaxation patio; twenty-four-hour fitness center

Special services: Two cabanas for outdoor massages, manicures, and pedicures

Signature treatment: Rollerssage Massage with semi-precious stones

Heavenly Spa by Westin

The Westin Maui Resort & Spa
2365 Kā'anapali Parkway
Kā'anapali, Hawai'i 96761
(808) 661-2588
www.westinmaui.com

Facility highlights: Sixteen treatment rooms, including two for couples that have a whirlpool; full-service beauty salon; men's and women's locker facilities with whirlpool, sauna, and steam rooms; open-air yoga/fitness studio; ocean-view relaxation lounge; manicure/

BELOW (CLOCKWISE FROM TOP LEFT): Infinity-edged soaking baths are among Spa Suites' amenities. Ingredients for Waikīkī Plantation Spa's treatments include (clockwise, from top) Hawaiian cane sugar with Ayurvedic herbs, a sugarcane scrub, a Kona coffee scrub, and Hawaiian sea salt with macadamia and *kukui* nut oils. Sunshine, fresh air, refreshments, and a spectacular view of the ocean lure guests to Waikīkī Plantation Spa's outdoor relaxation area.

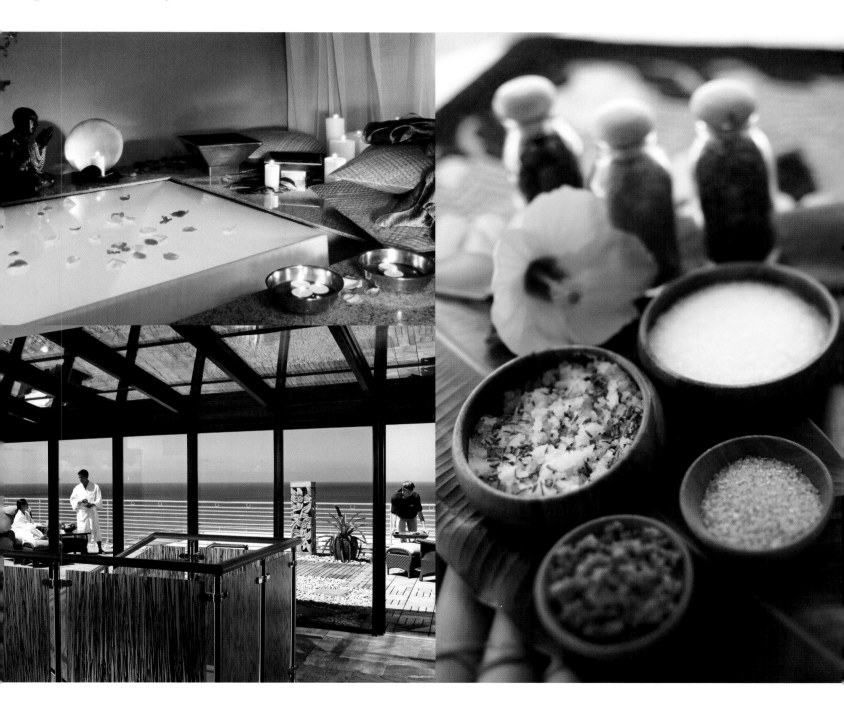

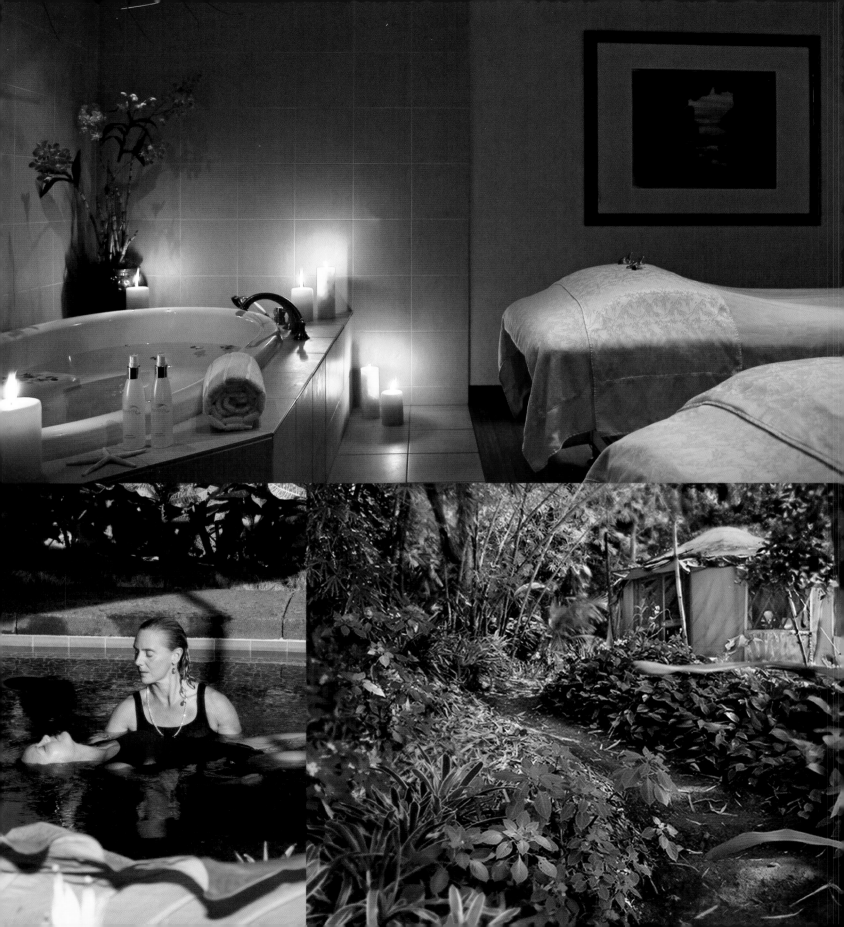

LEFT (CLOCKWISE FROM TOP): Heavenly Spa by Westin at The Westin Maui Resort & Spa has two treatment rooms for couples, each equipped with a whirlpool tub. At Luana Spa Retreat, treatments are performed in a yurt nestled among colorful flowers, verdant foliage, and tall stands of bamboo. Guests discover the healing power of water with Honua Spa's Aquatic Renewal treatment.

pedicure room for couples; twenty-four-hour fitness center; in-room spa services that include a gift basket filled with flowers, a CD of customized relaxation music, bottled water, and healthful treats

Special services: Partnership with Maui Lavender to create exclusive products for the spa's signature treatments

Signature treatment: Island Lavender Body Butter Treatment

Hina Mana Salon & Spa

The Whaler on Kā'anapali Beach
2481 Kā'anapali Parkway
Kā'anapali, Hawai'i 96761
(808) 661-7755
www.hinamana.com

Facility highlights: Three treatment rooms, including one for couples; sauna

Special services: The only full-service Aveda Concept Salon on Maui, it offers the complete line of Aveda products; wedding parties for up to ten people; pedicure bed; spa packages; therapists will travel anywhere on Maui for in-home treatments or in-room treatments at other hotels

Signature treatment: Clarity Boost with Lomilomi

Honua Spa

Hotel Hāna-Maui
5031 Hāna Highway
Hāna, Hawai'i 96713
(808) 270-5290
www.hotelhanamaui.com

Facility highlights: Nine treatment rooms, including two for couples; steam rooms; cold plunge pool; outdoor lava rock showers; Watsu pool; lava rock whirlpool; relaxation room in a beautifully landscaped low-rise bungalow set-

ting designed for an indoor/outdoor experience

Special services: Aquatic bodywork in Maui's only resort Watsu pool

Signature treatment: Hawaiian Lomilomi

Luana Spa Retreat

5050 Uakea Road
Hāna, Hawai'i 96713
(808) 248-8855
www.luanaspa.com

Facility highlights: Two yurts, one for overnight accommodations and one for spa treatments; a traditional Hawaiian *hale* for treatments and relaxation with a spectacular view of Hāna Bay; a covered, open-air gathering place to enjoy coffee drinks, teas, smoothies, sandwiches, wraps, and other healthful fare purchased at an on-site food cart

Special services: Lunch or candlelit dinner prepared by a personal chef for overnight or day spa guests; customized wedding packages, including overnight accommodations in the yurt, spa services for the couple, and ceremony and candlelit wedding dinner in the *hale*

Signature treatment: 'Awa 'Alaea Wrap

Makai Massage & Bodywork

Nāpili Kai Beach Resort
5900 Lower Honoapi'ilani Road
Nāpili, Hawai'i 96761

Facility highlights: Located oceanfront with two treatments rooms and a steam canopy

Special services: Spa packages, therapists will travel anywhere on Maui for in-home treatments or in-room treatments at other hotels

Signature treatment: Hāna Rainforest Wrap

Mandara Spa
Wailea Beach Marriott Resort & Spa
3700 Wailea Alanui
Wailea, Hawai'i 96753
(808) 891-8774
www.mandaraspa.com

Facility highlights: Twelve treatment rooms, oceanside cabana for massages, steam rooms in separate men's and women's relaxation lounges, full-service salon, fitness center

Special services: YSPA Teen Program with massages, facials, scrubs, and more

Signature treatment: Elemis Aroma Stone Therapy Massage

Spa at Black Rock
Sheraton Maui Resort
2605 Kā'anapali Parkway
Kā'anapali, Hawai'i 96761
(808) 661-0031
www.sheraton-maui.com

Facility highlights: Seven treatment rooms, including one couples' room with a soaking tub; three outdoor cabana treatment areas, including one for couples; three manicure stations; three pedicure stations; two indoor/outdoor relaxation areas

Special services: Custom packages, spa can be rented for private parties

Signature treatment: Pu'u Keka'a Stone Massage

Spa Grande
Grand Wailea Resort Hotel & Spa
3850 Wailea Alanui
Wailea, Hawai'i 96753
(808) 875-1234
www.grandwailea.com

Facility highlights: Fifty thousand square feet (the largest spa in Hawai'i); forty treatment rooms; one Family Spa Treatment Suite, where up to four members of a family can get a massage at the same time; two Spa Suites with tubs used for couples' treatments; relaxation lānai with ocean views

Special services: Complimentary Termé Wailea Hydrotherapy featuring Japanese furo bath, Roman tub, Swiss jet showers, cascading waterfall massage, and five specialty baths (Papaya Enzyme, 'Alaea Sea Salt, Limu Seaweed, Aromatherapy, and Moor Mud). Children's and teens' treatments such as Chocolate Coconut Massage; half-day Just for Men spa packages, some including the Volcanic Ash Purifying Facial and Hot Lava Stones Foot Treatment

Signature treatment: Six Hands Lava Stone Massage

Spa Kea Lani
The Fairmont Kea Lani, Maui
4100 Wailea Alanui
Wailea, Hawai'i 96753
(808) 875-2229
www.fairmont.com

Facility highlights: Nine treatment rooms, including one for couples

Special services: Poolside cabana massages

Signature treatment: Ala Lani Signature Body Experience

Spa Moana
Hyatt Regency Maui Resort & Spa
200 Nohea Kai Drive
Kā'anapali, Hawai'i 96761
(808) 667-4725
www.maui.hyatt.com

Facility highlights: Fifteen treatment rooms, including

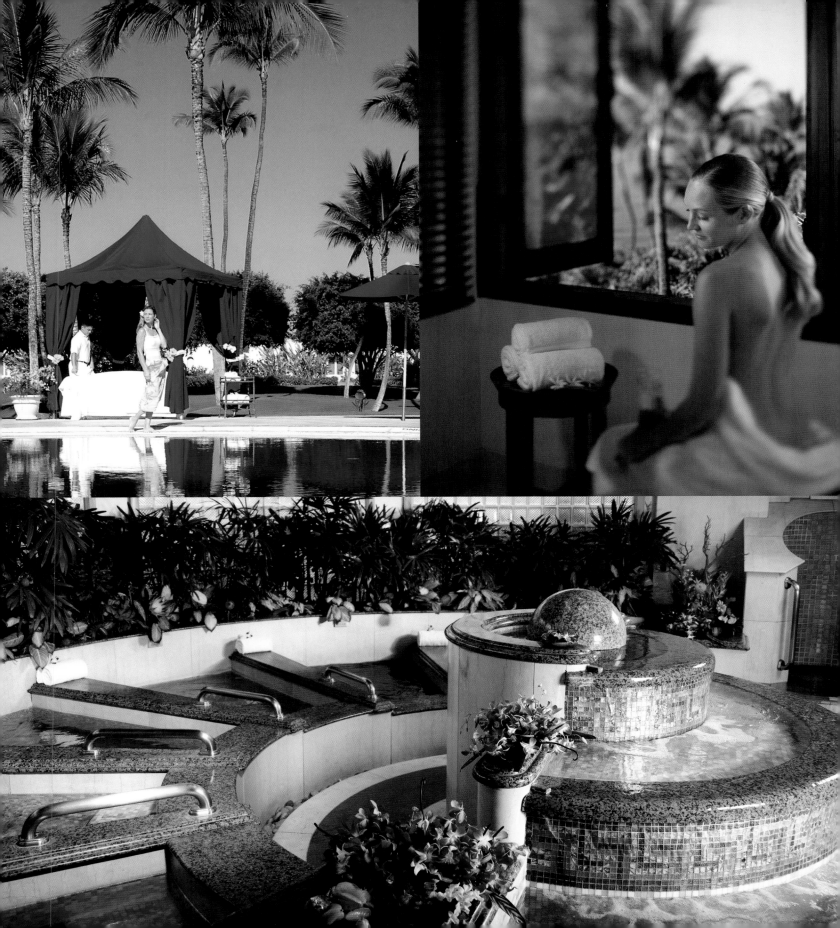

BELOW (CLOCKWISE FROM LEFT): Foot reflexology in an oceanfront spot is a popular option at The Spa at Four Seasons Resort Maui. Light pours into The Ritz-Carlton, Kapalua's fitness room through floor-to-ceiling windows. Spa Moana has two ocean-view suites for couples' treatments.

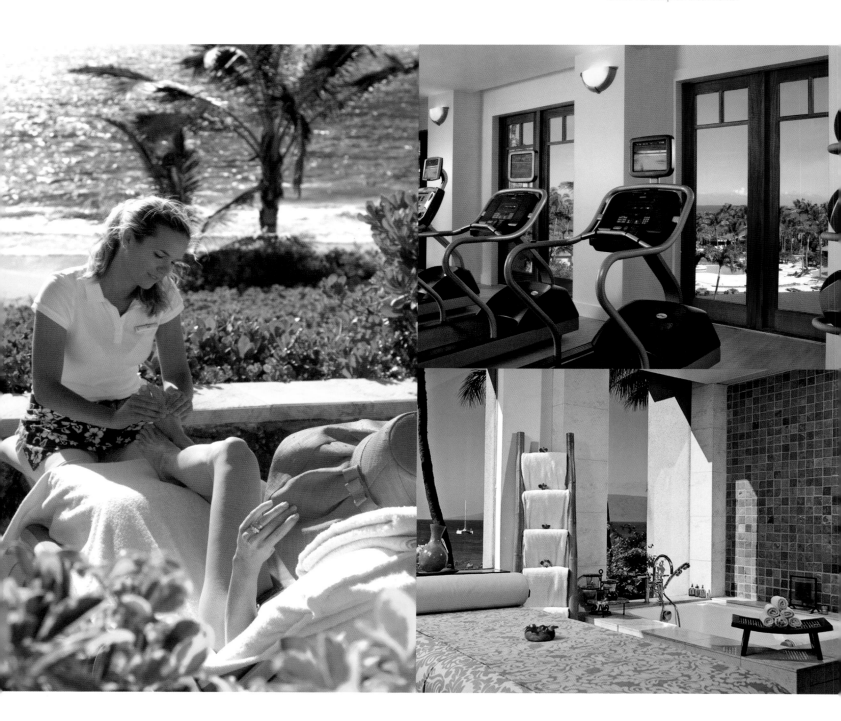

two spa suites for couples; steam rooms; saunas; whirl-pools; full-service salon overlooking the ocean; relaxation room; twenty-four-hour ocean-view athletic club with a dance/aerobic studio

Special services: Oceanside cabana massages, manicures, and pedicures; children's and teens' spa packages and yoga classes

Signature treatment: Hawaiian Pōhaku Treatment

The Ritz-Carlton Spa, Kapalua

The Ritz-Carlton, Kapalua
One Ritz-Carlton Drive
Kapalua, Hawai'i 96761
(808) 665-7280
www.ritzcarlton.com

Facility highlights: Fifteen treatment rooms, six opening to private outdoor shower gardens and two outdoor garden *hale* for couples; coed relaxation lounge with a whirlpool and outdoor Hawaiian garden; ocean-view fitness center; separate men's and women's relaxation lounges, each with saunas, steam rooms, rain showers, and whirlpools

Special services: Customized treatments for children, teenagers, and mothers-to-be

Signature treatment: Hawaiian Healing Experience

The Salon and Spa at Kā'anapali Shores

ResortQuest Kā'anapali Shores
3445 Lower Honoapi'ilani Road
Kā'anapali, Hawai'i 96761
(808) 661-0142
www.kshoresalonandspa.com

Facility highlights: Two treatment rooms, sauna, spa shower with hydromassage system, full-service salon

Special services: Wedding coordination, wedding and salon packages

Signature treatment: Mango and Mandarin Salt Scrub

The Spa at Four Seasons Resort Maui

Four Seasons Resort Maui at Wailea
3900 Wailea Alanui
Wailea, Hawai'i 96753
(808) 874-2925
www.fourseasons.com/maui

Facility highlights: Thirteen treatment rooms, including one for couples with a steam/rain shower and Jacuzzi; three oceanside *hale* for massages. The steam/rain shower is a "mini" steam room with a rain shower feature.

Special services: Massages in warm cocoon beds and a Tapas Spa Treatment menu that offers twenty-, thirty-, and forty-minute head, neck, shoulder, scalp, and foot massages poolside along with Evian spritzes; fruit kabobs; natural fruit Popsicles; chocolate and vanilla bean ice cream bars; iced bottled Evian; cucumber slices for your eyes; and chilled, scented face towels. Fitness offerings include Gyrotonics, which uses specially designed machines to emulate the movements of Pilates, *tai chi*, swimming, yoga, and gymnastics.

Signature treatment: E Ola Hou

RIGHT (CLOCKWISE FROM LEFT): *Pa'akai* (salt) is used for Hale Ho'ōla's signature treatment, Ma'ukele Volcano Rainforest 'Ike. Hawaiian *lomilomi* typically involves using the elbows. Here, a massage therapist at Hale Ho'ōla does that to relieve her client's sore muscles and to stimulate circulation. Walkways lined with graceful arches are among the architectural highlights of Ahu Pōhaku Ho'omaluhia.

Island of Hawai'i

A Beautiful Day Spa
16-1436 39th Street
Kea'au, Hawai'i 96749
(808) 982-7252
www.abeautifuldayspa.com

Facility highlights: Rainforest setting among eucalyptus, palms, tropical plants, and flowers; two indoor rooms and a garden gazebo for massage, all of which can accommodate couples' treatments; outdoor shower

Special services: Outdoor evening candlelight massage under the stars; complimentary daily "*lomi* yoga" class that combines traditional Hawaiian *lomilomi* and yoga techniques; accommodations in a treehouse and screened bamboo sleeping rooms; complimentary organic continental breakfast for guests booking stays

Signature treatment: Lomilomi Massage with Warm Stones

Ahu Pōhaku Ho'omaluhia
54-250 Lōkahi Road, Box 63
Hāwī, Hawai'i 96719
(808) 889-6336
www.hawaii-island-retreat.com

Facility highlights: Sixty-acre self-sustaining retreat with photovoltaic panels, windmills, and microhydro system; five private treatment *hale* large enough for couples for all services; three-hundred-square-foot guest rooms with soaking tubs; yoga studio; media room with big-screen TV and projection system for movies, presentations, and special programs; library with phones and Internet access; fruit, vegetable, and flower gardens with water features

Special services: Meditation classes, couples' retreats, weddings

Signature treatment: Maluhia

Big Island Spa & Tanning
29 Shipman Street, Suite 103
Hilo, Hawai'i 96720
(808) 961-1919
www.bigislandspatanning.com

Facility highlights: Seven treatment rooms, including an aromatherapeutic steam room and one for couples' massage; two rooms for aesthetic and beauty treatments, including facials, waxing, chemical peels, eyelash extensions, and eyebrow tinting

Special services: Wedding packages, indoor tanning

Signature treatment: Herbal and Natural Body Wrap

Hale Ho'ōla
Hawaiian Healing Arts Center and Spa
11-3913 Seventh Street
Volcano, Hawai'i 96785
(808) 756-2421
www.halehoola.net

Facility highlights: Suite large enough to accommodate couples, located in a tropical rainforest; outdoor reception area overlooking the rainforest

Special services: Hawaiian cultural workshops, steam canopy system (a massage table covered by a canopy that provides the benefits of a steam room)

Signature treatment: Ma'ukele Volcano Rainforest 'Ike

Ho'ōla Spa
Sheraton Keauhou Bay Resort & Spa
78-128 'Ehukai Street
Kailua-Kona, Hawai'i 96740
(808) 930-4848
www.sheratonkeauhou.com

Facility highlights: Seven treatment rooms, including one with a Vichy shower, one with a hot tub, and two for

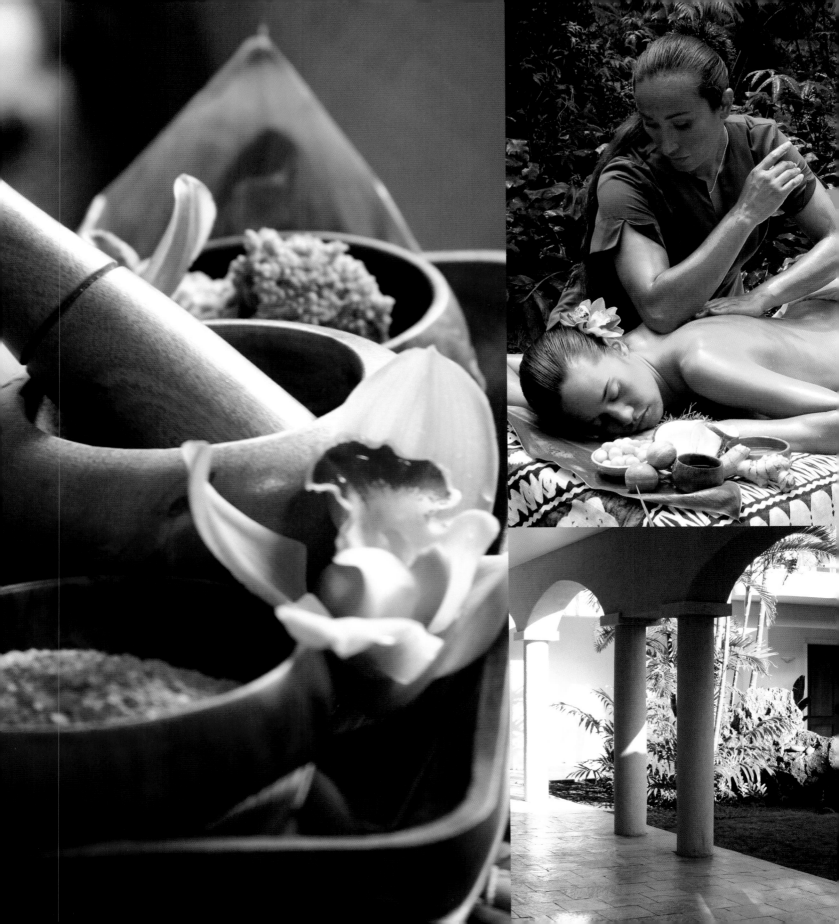

BELOW (CLOCKWISE FROM TOP LEFT): Guests at Ho'ōla Spa can have their massage treatments outdoors. Hualālai Sports Club & Spa offers eight thatched-roof *hale* for treatments. Mini waterfalls and brightly colored plants and blossoms create a lovely ambience at Kona Village Spa.

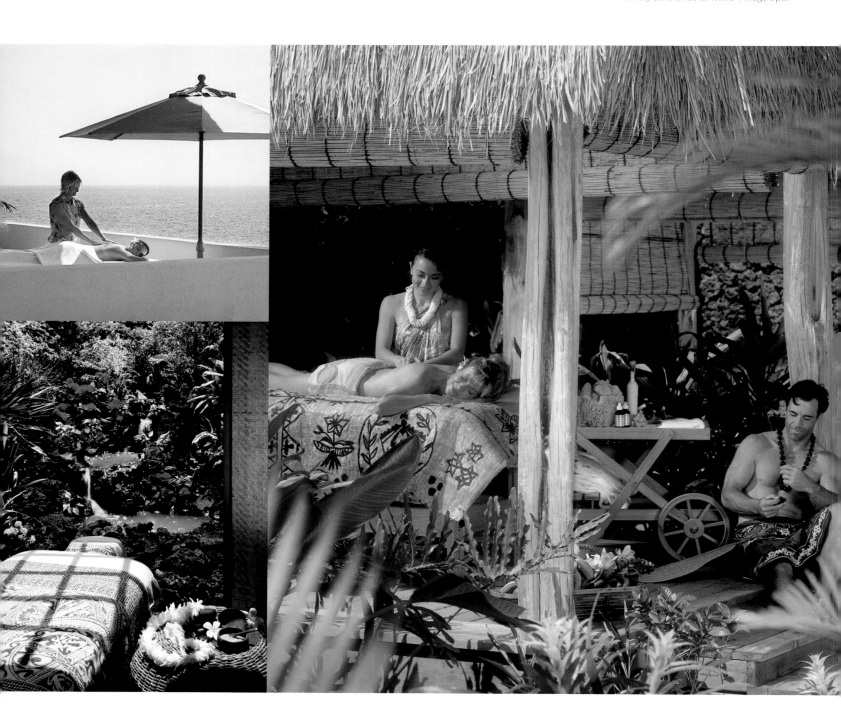

couples; steam room; outdoor infrared sauna; full-service salon overlooking the ocean and sea cliffs of Kona

Special services: Acupuncture, wedding packages

Signature treatment: Ho'ola Beaubelle Signature Body Treatment

Hualālai Sports Club & Spa

Four Seasons Resort Hualālai
100 Ka'ūpūlehu Drive
Kailua-Kona, Hawai'i 96740
(808) 325-8440
www.fourseasons.com/hualalai/vacations/spa_services.html

Facility highlights: Sixteen treatment rooms, including eight outdoor *hale* and one outdoor facial area; steam rooms; saunas; lap pool; indoor/outdoor showers; beauty salon; open-air yoga studio; half-court basketball court

Special services: Climbing classes on a custom-designed twenty-four-foot-high outdoor wall; ocean programs, including canoe paddling, ocean swims, and surfing lessons

Signature treatment: Polynesian Niu Scrub

Kālona Salon & Spa

Outrigger Keauhou Beach Resort
78-6740 Ali'i Drive
Kailua-Kona, Hawai'i 96740
(808) 322-9373
www.kalonaspa.com

Facility highlights: An oceanside outdoor garden area accommodating one or two people, two indoor treatment rooms, full-service salon

Special services: Specialized services for brides, couples, children, teens, moms-to-be, and men, including Sports Pedicure (men) and Facial/Pedicure with nail jewelry (teens)

Signature treatment: Kālona Pōhaku Healing Stone Massage

Kohala Sports Club & Spa

Hilton Waikoloa Village
425 Waikoloa Beach Drive
Waikoloa, Hawai'i 96738
(808) 886-2828
www.kohalaspa.com

Facility highlights: Twenty-four treatment rooms, including three for couples' massages; four private whirlpool baths; cardiovascular and weight rooms; sauna; steam room; indoor/outdoor garden with whirlpool; relaxation lounges; full-service salon

Special services: Personal training, movement therapy

Signature treatment: Orchid Isle Massage

Kona Village Spa

Kona Village Resort
P.O. Box 1299
Kailua-Kona, Hawai'i 96745
(808) 325-5555
www.konavillage.com

Facility highlights: Four indoor/outdoor treatment rooms, each with an adjacent changing room with sauna and shower, and a waterfall providing soothing ambient sounds; adjacent open-air fitness center

Special services: In-*hale* and oceanside massages (including a couple's *hale*), nutrition and personal fitness training

Signature treatment: Limu Healing Body Mask with Peppermint Scrub

RIGHT (CLOCKWISE FROM LEFT): A massage *hale* at Spa Without Walls sits over a waterfall. The sun heats a lava sauna at Mauna Lani Spa. Concoctions at Paul Brown Salon & Spa at Hāpuna include ingredients such as green seaweed, chocolate, macadamia nuts, and pineapple. Happiness is a facial at Mandara Spa at Waikoloa Resort.

Mandara Spa

Waikoloa Beach Marriott Resort & Spa
69-275 Waikoloa Beach Drive
Waikoloa, Hawai'i 96738
(808) 886-8191
www.mandaraspa.com

Facility highlights: Seven treatment rooms, including two for couples; steam rooms in separate men's and women's relaxation lounges; full-service salon

Special services: YSPA Teen Program with massages, facials, scrubs, and more; CustomBronzing Spray Tanning

Signature treatment: Elemis Aroma Spa Ocean Detox Wrap

Mauna Lani Spa

Mauna Lani Resort
68-1365 Pauoa Road
Kohala Coast, Hawai'i 96743
(808) 881-7922
www.maunalani.com

Facility highlights: Outdoor thatched *hale* for treatments, all with outdoor showers (two are large enough for couples, two have lava rock tubs for specialty treatments, and one has an outdoor Vichy shower); two naturally heated lava saunas; *lā'au* garden; outdoor open-air relaxation pavilion overlooking the garden; Watsu pool set within a lava tube; eight indoor treatment rooms, including one for couples with a steam shower and whirlpool bath; saunas; steam rooms; fitness area including an aerobics room; outdoor whirlpool; twenty-five-meter lap pool

Special services: Private wedding parties or meeting events in a Hawaiian village setting

Signature treatment: Lava Watsu

Paul Brown Salon & Spa at Hāpuna

Hāpuna Beach Prince Hotel
62-100 Kauna'oa Drive
Kohala Coast, Hawai'i 96743
(808) 880-3335
www.paulbrownhawaii.com

Facility highlights: Seven treatment rooms, two saunas and steam rooms, two manicure/pedicure stations, one makeup station, four hairdressing stations, four outdoor massage cabanas

Special services: Traditional Chinese therapies, including acupuncture and herbal medicine

Signature treatment: Hāpuna Pele Experience

Spa Without Walls

Fairmont Orchid Hawai'i
One North Kanikū Drive
Kohala Coast, Hawai'i 96743
(808) 887-7540
www.fairmont.com

Facility highlights: Ten massage *hale* set among waterfalls and streams, including one for couples; five oceanfront massage cabanas, all accommodating couples; three indoor treatment rooms; steam room; sauna; full-service salon; fitness center

Special services: Two of the waterfall *hale*, cantilevered over the waterway, allow guests to view koi swimming beneath them during their treatment. Fitness and art classes include Awakening the Artist Within, Drawing in Nature, and Vision and Memory Fitness (the basics of maintaining and improving your eyesight and memory naturally)

Signature treatment: Hawai'i's Big Island Kona Coffee Vanilla Exfoliation Treatment

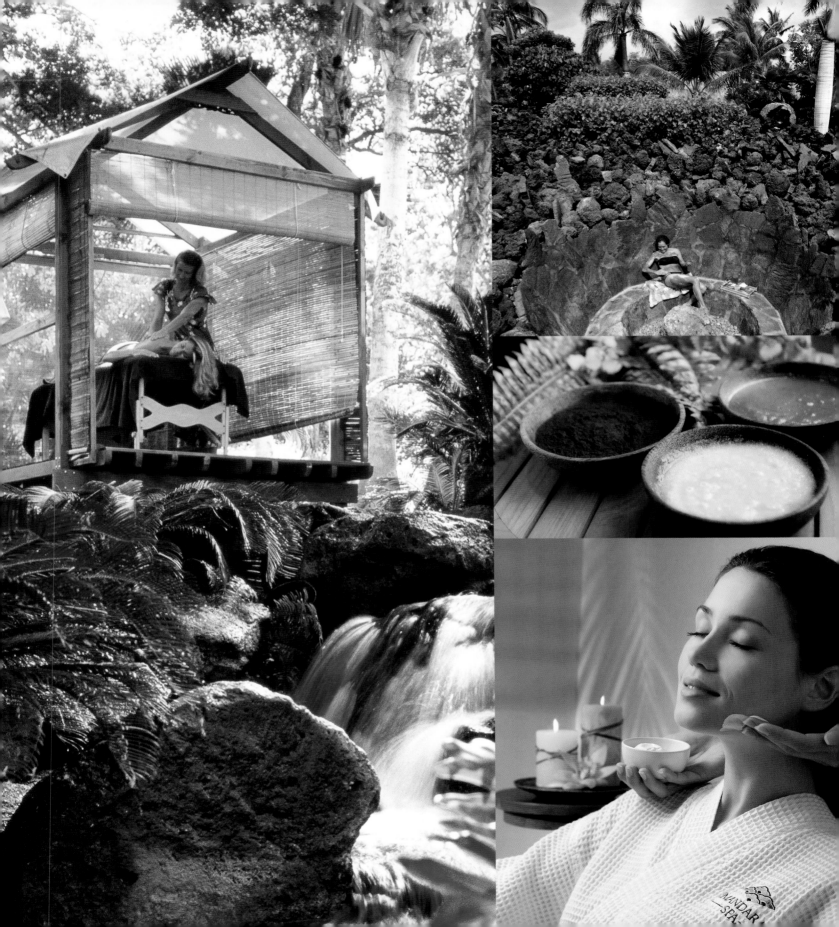

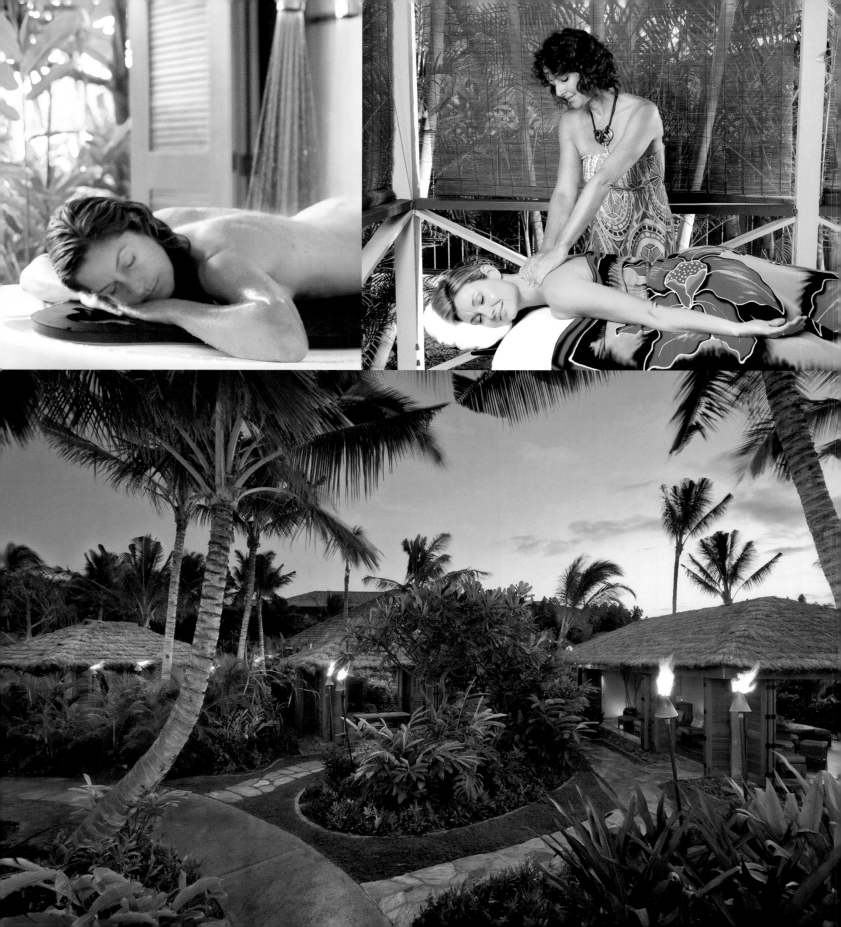

LEFT (CLOCKWISE FROM BOTTOM): Torches light Anara Spa's Lōkahi Garden, which is comprised of five treatment *hale* and a relaxation *hale*. One of Anara Spa's treatment rooms is designated for Vichy showers. A guest relishes the magic of a massage at A Hideaway Spa.

Kaua'i

A Hideaway Spa

ResortQuest Waimea Plantation Cottages
9400 Kaumuali'i Highway
Waimea, Hawai'i 96796
(808) 338-0005
www.ahideawayspa.com

Facility highlights: Three treatment rooms; wet room; *lānai* space for couples' massages; full-service salon; spa boutique; steam room; hydrotherapy tub; two plantation-style cottages and their surrounding gardens used as outdoor treatment and relaxation areas

Special services: Customized packages; beachfront yoga classes; makeup applications for weddings, proms, and other special occasions; pedicures using pipe-free Jacuzzi tub (no recirculation of water) and roller and vibration massage chair; products handmade with organic ingredients such as kava, blossoms, honey, seaweed, and citrus; wraps and scrubs are locally made exclusively for A Hideaway Spa

Signature treatment: Lomilomi 'Ili'ili Massage

Alexander Day Spa and Salon

Kaua'i Marriott Resort and Beach Club
3610 Rice Street, Suite 9A
Līhu'e, Kaua'i 96766
(808) 246-4918
www.alexanderspa.com

Facility highlights: Four treatment rooms, including one for couples; two beachside massage cabanas; full-service salon

Special services: Wedding and bridal packages

Signature treatment: Pūholo Steam Canopy and Massage

Anara Spa

Grand Hyatt Kaua'i Resort & Spa
1571 Po'ipū Road
Po'ipū, Hawai'i 96756
(808) 240-6440
www.anaraspa.com

Facility highlights: Eight indoor/outdoor massage rooms opening to their own private gardens; five outdoor treatment *hale* (including two for couples) with private tropical grottoes and lava rock shower areas; three indoor/outdoor facial rooms; two botanical soaking tubs; one Vichy room; two indoor steam rooms and saunas; twenty-five-yard lap pool; twenty-four-hour fitness center

Special services: Lōkahi Garden, where the treatment *hale* are, may be rented for private parties

Signature treatment: Kaua'i Clay Ritual

Hanalei Day Spa

Hanalei Colony Resort
5-7132 Kūhiō Highway
Hanalei, Hawai'i 96714
(808) 826-6621
www.hanaleidayspa.com

Facility highlights: Four treatment rooms, including two for couples (one is beachside)

Special services: Private ladies' spa party; healing retreats; customized yoga sessions; Massages of the World, from Ayurveda to Zen Shiatsu

Signature treatment: Pancha Karma

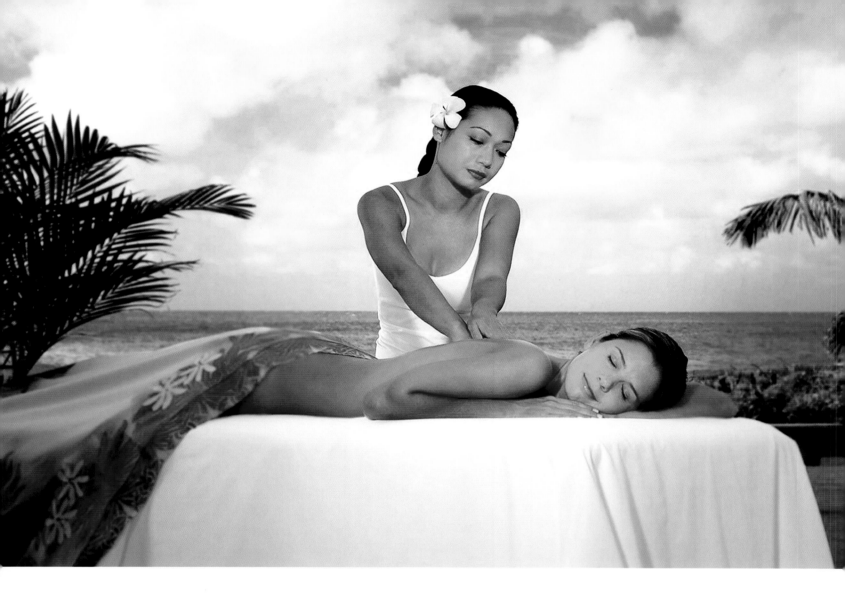

Hawaiian Rainforest Salon & Spa

Hilton Kaua'i Beach Resort
4331 Kaua'i Beach Drive
Līhu'e, Hawai'i 96766
(808) 246-5529
www.hawaiianrainforest.com

Facility highlights: Four treatment rooms (two of them for couples), gym, sauna, hair salon with pedicure spa

Special services: Exclusive use in the United States of Beaubelle products from Switzerland

Signature treatment: Body Elixir Trio

Pua Day Spa

ResortQuest Kaua'i Beach at Makaiwa
650 Aleka Loop
Kapa'a, Hawai'i 96746
www.hawaiianrainforest.com

Facility highlights: One treatment room that can accommodate couples, hair salon, pedicure spa, furnishings and flooring imported from Bali

Special services: Owned and operated by Hawaiian Rainforest Salon & Spa, the company that has exclusive use in the United States of Beaubelle products from Switzerland

Signature treatment: Slimming and Detoxifying Body Wrap

LEFT: Your worries will
melt away at The Stylists
Salon & Massage Center.

"SPA"CIAL HAVENS | 153

The Stylists Salon & Massage Center

Sheraton Kaua'i Resort
2440 Hoonoani Road
Po'ipū, Hawai'i 96756
(808) 742-4038
www.hawaiianrainforest.com

Facility highlights: Two treatment rooms, oceanfront cabana

Special services: Customized facials; owned and operated by Hawaiian Rainforest Salon & Spa, the company that has exclusive use in the United States of Beaubelle products from Switzerland

Signature treatment: Na Lani Mea

Waipouli Beach Resort Spa and Salon Aveda

Outrigger Waipouli Beach Resort & Spa
4-820 Kūhiō Highway, Suite 3
Kapa'a, Hawai'i 96746
(808) 823-1488

Facility highlights: Four treatment rooms; one Vichy shower room; five poolside cabanas for massage, one for couples

Special services: Hawai'i's first and only resort spa with the Aveda Lifestyle designation, meaning Aveda products are used for all treatments; some packages include $10 vouchers for products sold in the spa's shop

Signature treatment: Elemental Nature Massage

Moloka'i

Hotel Moloka'i Spa Center

Hotel Moloka'i
1300 Kamehameha V Highway
Kaunakakai, Hawai'i 96748
(808) 660-3334
www.hotelmolokai.com

Facility highlights: One treatment room

Special services: Beachside yoga classes

Signature treatment: Lomilomi Massage and Facial

Lāna'i

The Spa

Four Seasons Resort Lāna'i at Mānele Bay
One Mānele Bay Road
Lāna'i City, Hawai'i 96763
(808) 565-2088
www.fourseasons.com/spa

Facility highlights: Ten treatment rooms, one outdoor garden *hale*, red cedar saunas, eucalyptus steam rooms, full-service salon, rainforest showers (seated stalls with ten-inch showerheads that provide a massage and create the sensation of being beneath a waterfall)

Special services: The spa can be reserved after its regular hours of operation for private sessions.

Signature treatment: Tropical Bliss

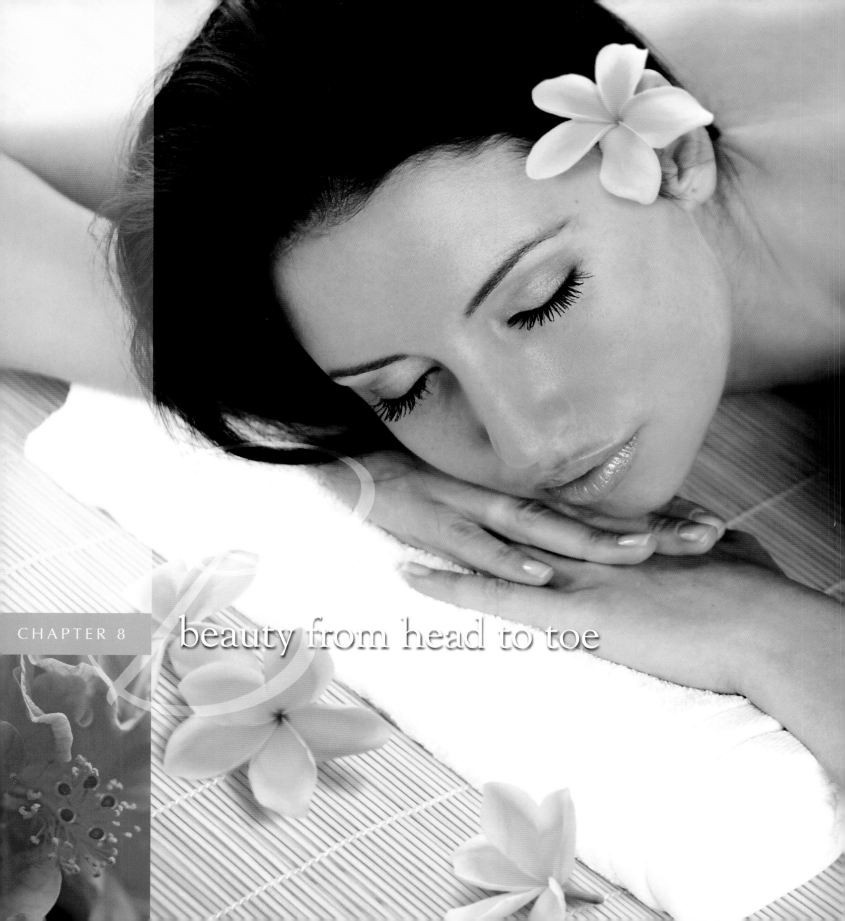

beauty from head to toe

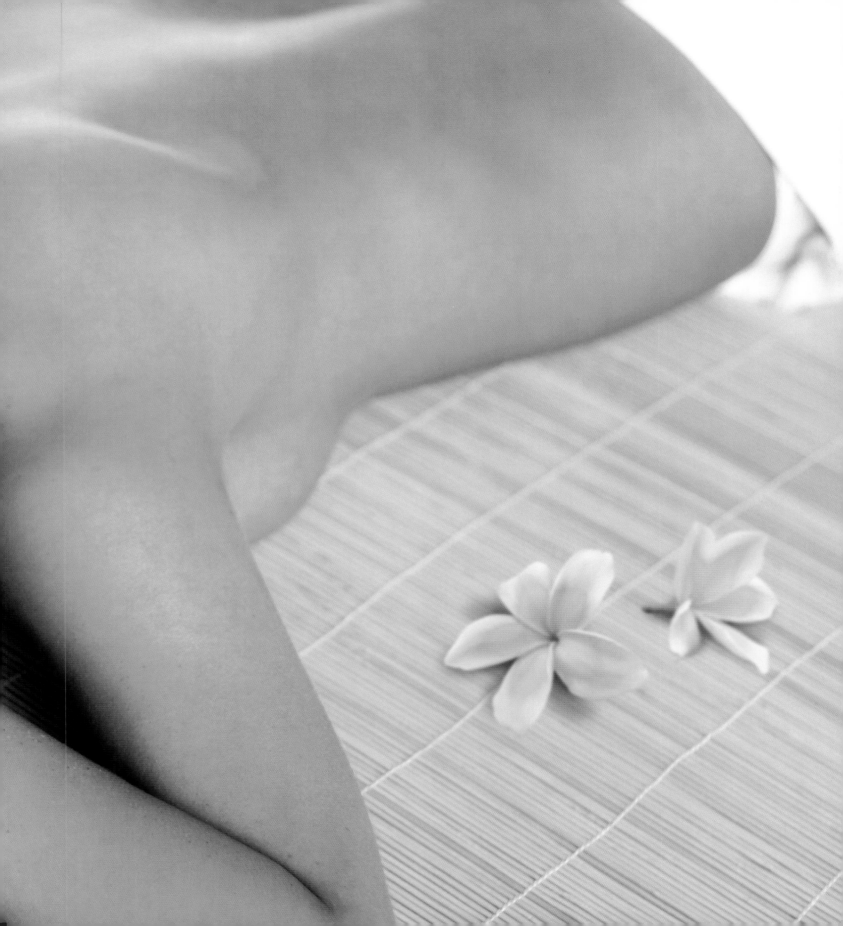

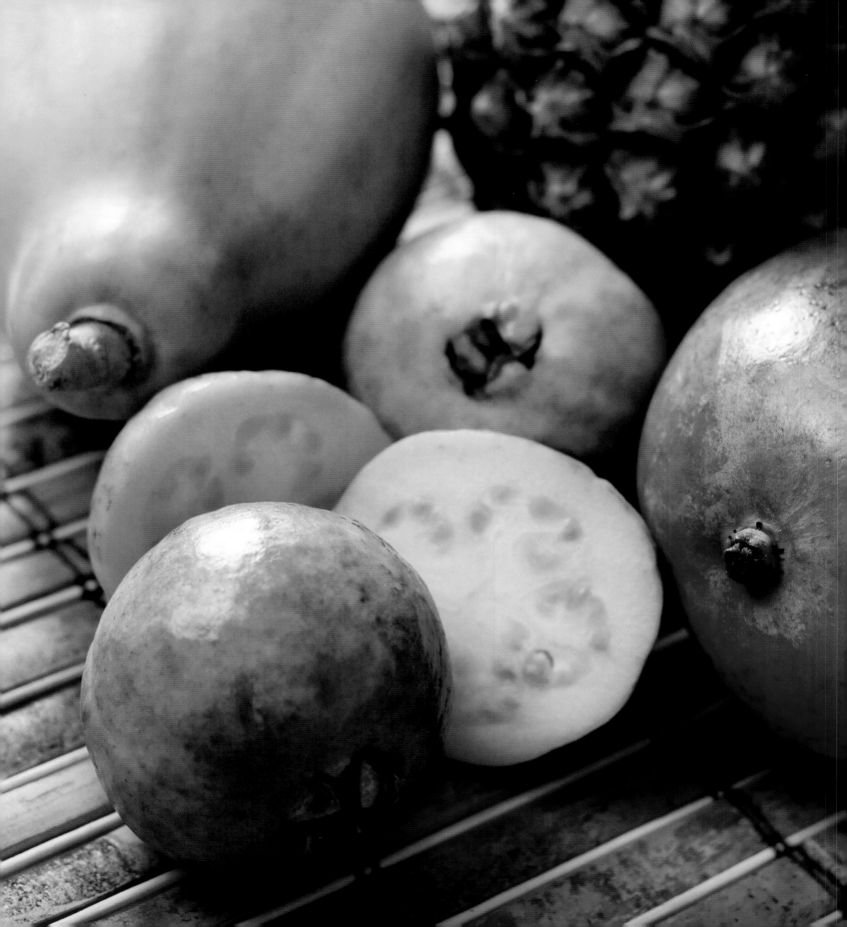

chapter 8

Look around your kitchen. Chances are you have everything you need to make these fifty delicious beauty recipes right at hand. Best of all, you don't have to be an accomplished cosmetologist to do so. All require just minutes of preparation time. First, ensure your ingredients are fresh. Don't use what you wouldn't put into your body onto your body.

Also, don't use tools and equipment with aluminum, silver, copper, Teflon, or cast-iron finishes, as contact with some ingredients may cause a reaction. Instead, opt for bowls, pots, jars, cups, and utensils made of glass, enameled clay, or stainless steel.

Finally, reserve a day when you won't be disturbed to make and try these treatments; that's the only way you'll enjoy optimum results. Close the door and open your mind. Turn off your phones and turn on some calming music. Now . . . indulge!

PRECEDING SPREAD: Make your own beauty products for relaxing spa experiences at home.

LEFT: Fresh fruits are the foundations for homemade lotions, shampoos, masks, and more.

FOR THE BODY

Banana Moisturizer

½   banana, peeled
1   tsp. honey
1   Tbsp. heavy whipping cream
1   drop chamomile essential oil
1   Tbsp. finely ground oatmeal (more if the consistency of the mixture is too runny, less if it's too thick)

Mash banana. Warm honey and whipping cream in microwave for about 15 seconds and stir to combine. Add to banana and mix well. Add chamomile oil and oatmeal and mix again. Apply to dampened skin with gentle, sweeping motions. Leave on for a few minutes. Rinse.

RIGHT: Orange juice is one of just three ingredients in the Sweet Body Scrub (see recipe on this page).

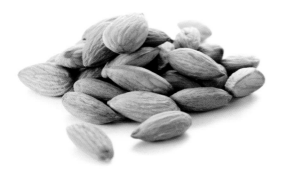

Almond Exfoliant

⅔   c. ground almonds
⅓   c. oatmeal
½   tsp. dried herbs of your choice
Plain yogurt, milk, or buttermilk (enough to make a paste)

Blend dry ingredients until the consistency of coarse meal. Store in a screw-top glass jar in refrigerator. When ready to use, scoop ¼ cup of dried mixture into a small bowl and stir in enough yogurt, milk, or buttermilk to make a paste. Rub paste on body. Rinse.

Milk and Citrus Peel Soak

1   c. powdered milk
¼   c. coarsely chopped orange peels
¼   c. coarsely chopped lemon peels
4   drops lavender essential oil

Draw a warm bath. While water is flowing, slowly add ingredients into tub. Mix well. Soak in bath for 20 minutes.

Sweet Body Scrub

½   c. brown sugar
Juice ½ orange
1   Tbsp. vitamin E oil

Mix ingredients. Dampen skin and apply mixture with gentle circular motions. Rinse.

Coconut Curry Mask

1   c. coconut milk
2   c. oatmeal
⅔   c. sweet almond oil
⅓   c. curry powder

Blend ingredients until the consistency of paste. Apply to body. Leave on for 20 minutes. Rinse.

Macadamia Cleansing Grains

2   c. oatmeal
½   c. unsalted macadamia nuts
2   Tbsp. dried rose petals
2   Tbsp. dried lavender flowers
Warm water (enough to make a paste)
½   tsp. almond oil (optional)

Finely grind each dry ingredient in separate batches. Mix together well and store in a covered container in a cool, dry place. To use, mix 1 heaping teaspoon of cleansing grains with enough warm water to make a creamy paste. If you have dry skin, add almond oil. Gently massage mixture onto your skin. Rinse with warm water.

Ginger, Lemon, and Parsley Bath

¼   c. minced fresh ginger root
½   c. grated lemon peel
¼   c. dried parsley
2   Tbsp. oatmeal

Mix ingredients. Put in a muslin cloth and tie at the top, forming a little bag. Attach cloth to the bathtub faucet as you draw a warm bath so that the running water goes through it, or place bag directly in tub. Soak in bath for 20 minutes.

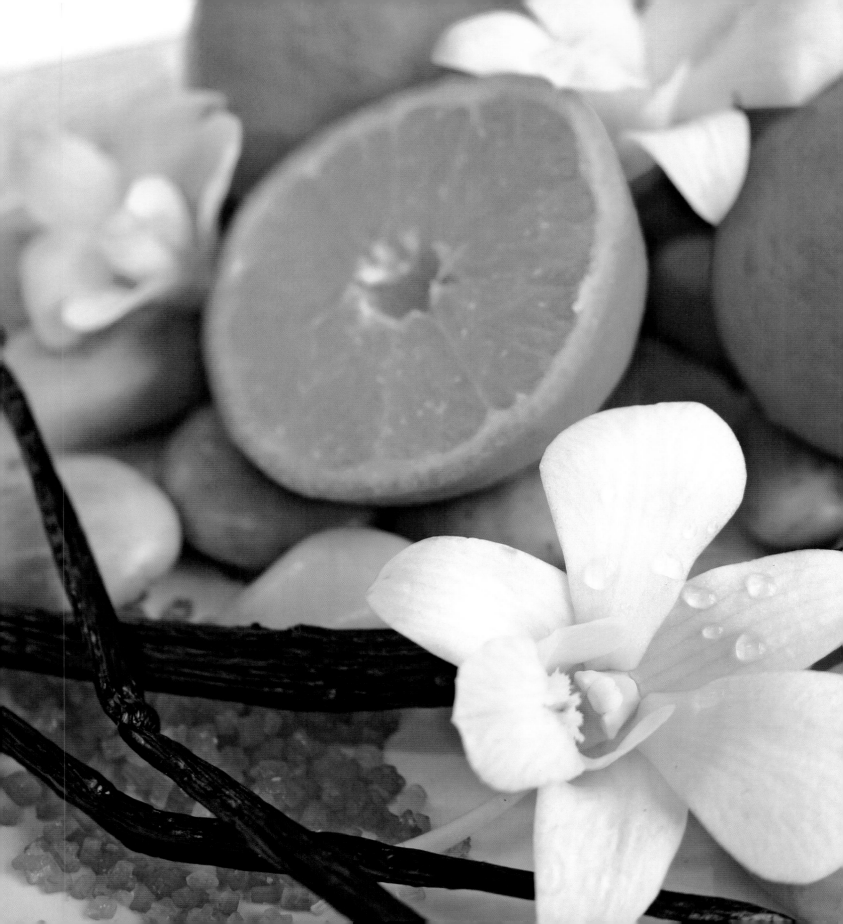

RIGHT: Facial creams, including Blueberry Balm (see recipe on facing page), should be applied with upward, circular motions.

Rainbow in a Jar

3 packets unflavored unsweetened Kool-Aid (one each of 3 different colors)
12 c. coarse sea salt
3–4 drops essential oils that complement the Kool-Aid flavors (i.e., orange oil with orange Kool-Aid, lavender oil with grape Kool-Aid, peppermint oil with strawberry Kool-Aid, etc.)

Mix 1 packet of Kool-Aid with 4 cups of salt; mix the 3 different colors in separate bowls. Add a corresponding essential oil to each bowl. Alternate colored layers in a glass or plastic container for storage. To use, add ½ to 1 cup of salts per bath. Note: The Kool-Aid will not stain your skin or tub, as it will be in fairly small concentrations, but be aware it could stain light-colored towels.

Kona Coffee Rub

2 c. coarsely ground Kona coffee
½ c. raw sugar
3 Tbsp. olive oil

Mix ingredients well. Take a hot shower to moisten skin and open pores. Using wide, circular motions, rub coffee exfoliant on your body with strong, even pressure. Rinse.

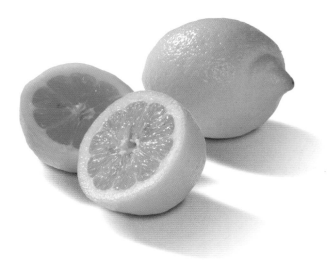

Fresh Fruit Salad

2 slices pineapple, rind removed
½ medium honeydew melon, rind removed
12 green grapes
1 medium banana, peeled
1 medium pear, cored
1 medium kiwi, peeled

Purée ingredients (the mixture will be slightly lumpy). Refrigerate 1 hour. Apply to body. Leave on for 30 minutes. Rinse with warm water.

Coconut and Tea Bath

1 c. oatmeal
1 c. brown rice
1 tsp. coconut extract
Contents 5 black tea bags
1 c. powdered milk

Mix ingredients, then divide in half. Cut 2 8-inch squares of cheesecloth and put half of mixture into each square. Tie at the top, forming pouches. Put 1 pouch in bath under running water and save the other for later use. Soak in bath for 20 minutes.

Honey-Lemon Lotion

1 tsp. honey
1 tsp. vegetable oil
¼ tsp. lemon juice

Mix ingredients. Apply to dry areas on skin. Leave on for 10 minutes. Rinse with warm water.

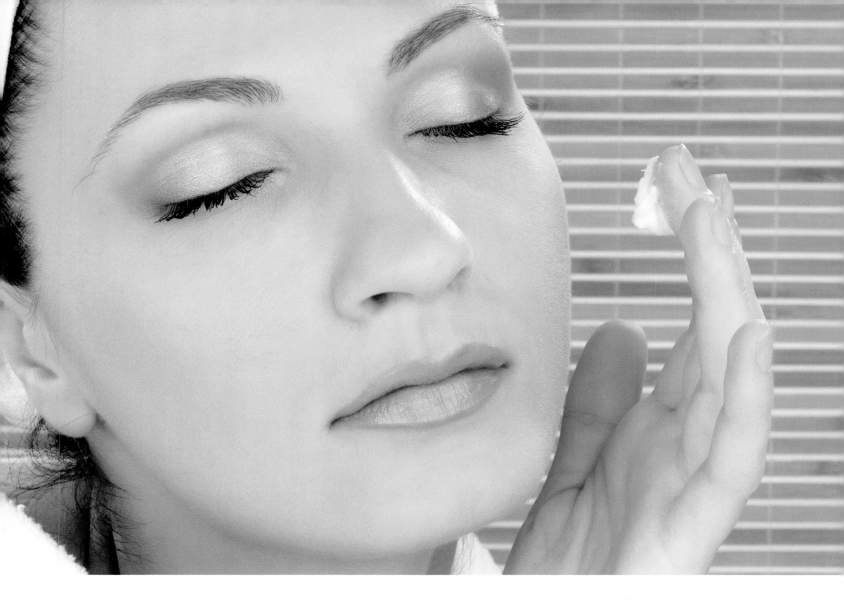

Yogurt Body Mask

3   Tbsp. puréed cooked pumpkin or carrots
     (canned also can be used)
¼   c. yogurt
3   Tbsp. honey

Mix pumpkin or carrots with yogurt and honey. Lather body with mask. Draw a warm bath and soak in it for 20 minutes.

FOR THE FACE

Blueberry Balm

1   c. plain yogurt
½   avocado, peeled, seeded, and mashed
10   blueberries, mashed
1   tsp. vanilla extract
2   tsp. ground cinnamon

Blend yogurt, avocado, and blueberries until smooth. Add vanilla extract and cinnamon and mix well. Massage over face and neck. Leave on for 15 minutes. Rinse using a warm washcloth.

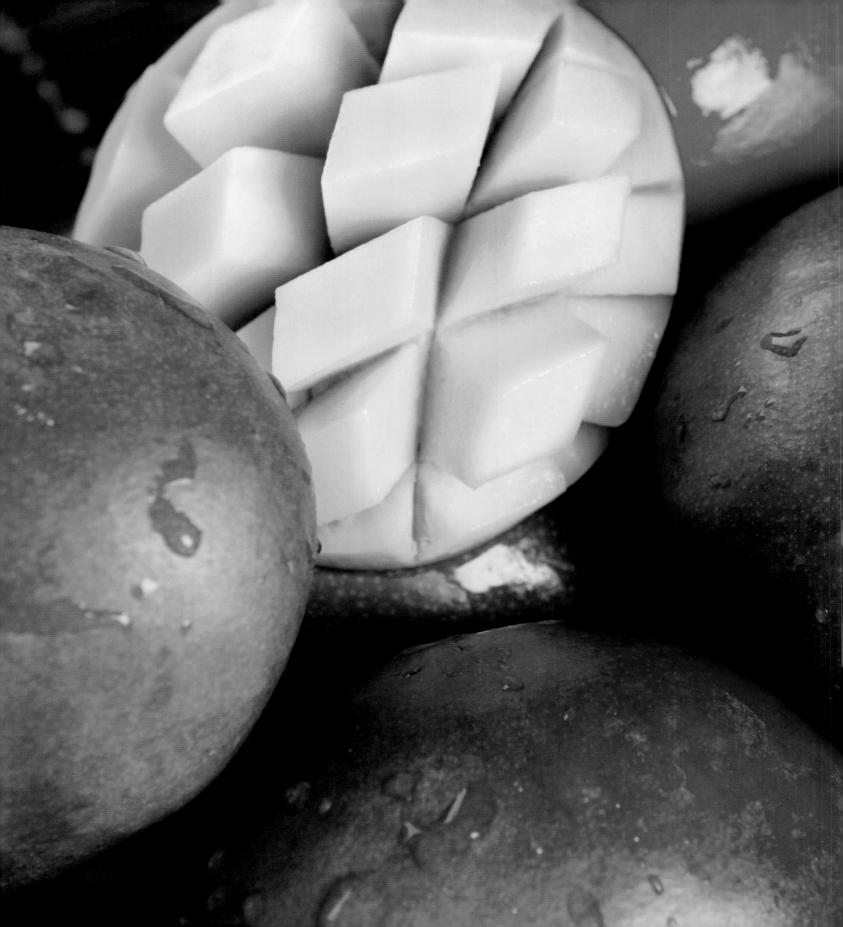

Cucumber Antiwrinkle Cream

½	cucumber, unpeeled
1	egg white
2	Tbsp. mayonnaise
½	c. wheat germ, olive, or avocado oil

Wash cucumber. Cube and blend with remaining ingredients. Apply to face and neck. Leave on for 10 minutes. Wipe off and follow with your normal cleansing regimen. For optimum results, use twice daily, in the morning and evening.

Chocolate Truffle

⅓	c. cocoa powder
3	Tbsp. heavy whipping cream
2	tsp. cottage cheese
¼	c. honey
3	tsp. powdered oatmeal

Mix ingredients. Smooth onto face. Leave on for 10 minutes, then rinse with warm water.

Papaya Peel

1	packet unflavored gelatin
3	Tbsp. distilled water
1	papaya, peeled and seeded

In a saucepan, combine gelatin and water. Warm over low heat until gelatin dissolves. Purée papaya. Strain out solids and reserve papaya juice in a small bowl. Add gelatin to juice. Refrigerate for about 20 minutes or until gelatin starts to set. Spread mixture over face and neck. Leave on for 15 minutes. Rinse with a soft sponge or towel dipped in warm water.

Mango Magic

¼	medium mango, peeled and seeded
2	Tbsp. oatmeal, finely powdered
2	Tbsp. almonds, finely powdered
2	Tbsp. heavy whipping cream (use whole milk if your skin is not dry)
	Distilled water (as needed; optional)

Blend ingredients for 1 minute, until mixture is smooth and creamy. (If it is too thick to spread on skin, add a bit of distilled water; if too runny, add more oatmeal.) Apply to face and neck. Leave on for 15 minutes. Rinse.

Grapefruit Refresher

1	egg white
1	tsp. sour cream
1	tsp. grapefruit juice

Beat egg white until fluffy. Add sour cream and grapefruit juice and blend well. Apply to face. Leave on for 15 minutes. Rinse with warm water.

Watermelon Astringent

2	Tbsp. fresh watermelon juice
1	Tbsp. vodka
2	Tbsp. witch hazel
2	Tbsp. distilled water

Strain watermelon juice to remove seeds and fruit pieces. Combine with other ingredients and stir well. Put mixture in a clean container with a tight-fitting lid. To use, pour a small amount on a clean cotton pad and apply to face. Store in refrigerator between uses to retain freshness. Will keep about 1 week.

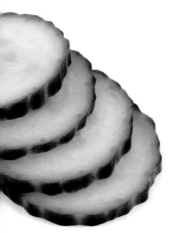

Cucumber and Tea Mask

1	small cucumber, peeled and seeded
4	Tbsp. green tea, steeped and strained
4	Tbsp. chamomile tea, steeped and strained
1	packet unflavored gelatin
2	Tbsp. aloe vera gel

Purée cucumber until smooth. Strain purée and reserve juice. In a small saucepan, combine teas and gelatin. Stir over low heat until gelatin is dissolved. Remove from heat and pour into a glass bowl. Add cucumber juice and aloe gel. Refrigerate for about 25 minutes, until mixture starts to thicken. Spread over face and neck. Allow to dry for 20 minutes. Peel off mask and rinse with warm water.

Thyme and Fennel Cleanser

2	sprigs fresh or ½ Tbsp. dried thyme, crumbled
2	tsp. whole fennel seeds, crushed
½	c. boiling water
	Juice ½ lemon

Mix thyme and fennel seeds. Cover with boiling water. Add lemon juice and steep for 15 minutes. Strain, pouring liquid in a jar. Refrigerate liquid until ready to use. Dab on face and neck with a cotton ball. Rinse.

Avocado and Carrot Cream

1	avocado, peeled, seeded, and mashed
1	carrot, cooked and mashed
½	c. heavy whipping cream
1	egg, beaten
3	Tbsp. honey

Blend ingredients until smooth. Spread over face and neck. Leave on for 15 minutes. Rinse with cool water.

Apple-Pear Wrinkle Fighter

1	tsp. apple juice
1	tsp. lemon juice
1	tsp. lime juice
2	Tbsp. buttermilk
1	Tbsp. fresh or dried rosemary leaves
3	seedless grapes
¼	pear, skinned and cored
2	egg whites

Blend ingredients on medium speed for 30 seconds. Cover and refrigerate immediately. To use, dab mixture on face with a cotton ball. Let dry, then rinse with warm water and apply moisturizer. Use no more than 3 times a week. Will keep in refrigerator for 4 days.

Facial Piña Colada

¼	c. fresh pineapple, peeled and finely chopped
1	Tbsp. coconut milk

Blend ingredients until smooth. Spread in a thin layer on face. Leave on for 10 minutes. Rinse with warm water.

Papaya-Strawberry Treat

1	Tbsp. oatmeal
½	ripe papaya, peeled and seeded
4	strawberries, stemmed
1	tsp. honey
1	tsp. fresh lemon juice

Grind oatmeal until powdered. Set aside. Cube papaya and strawberries; blend until smooth. Set aside. Warm honey gently until it flows freely; do not boil it. In a small bowl, combine ingredients with lemon juice and mix well. Apply to face. Leave on for 15 minutes. Rinse with warm water.

RIGHT: Sugar and cinnamon imbue the Cinnamon-Sugar Scrub with a wonderful fragrance (see recipe on this page).

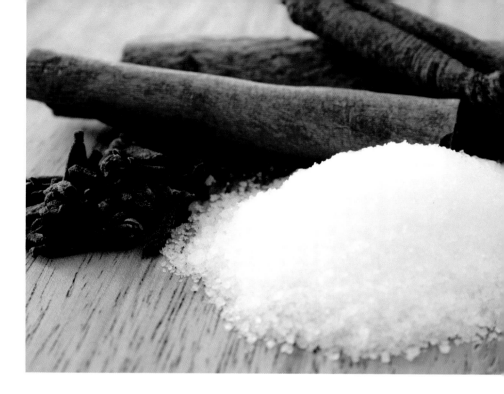

FOR THE HANDS AND FEET

Pumpkin Pie

3 Tbsp. canned pumpkin
1 Tbsp. brown sugar
2 Tbsp. olive oil
1 drop vanilla extract

Thoroughly mix ingredients. Gently massage mixture on hands and feet. Leave on for 10 minutes. Rinse with warm water.

Avocado Manicure

¼ avocado, peeled, seeded, and mashed
1 egg white
2 Tbsp. oatmeal
1 tsp. lemon juice

Blend ingredients into a paste. Apply to hands. Leave on for 20 minutes. Rinse with warm water.

Strawberry Soother

8–10 strawberries, stemmed
2 Tbsp. olive oil
1 tsp. coarse kosher or sea salt

Mix ingredients. Massage on hands and feet. Rinse.

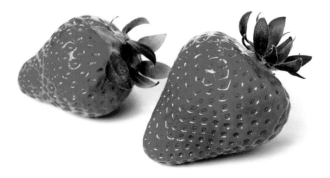

Overnight Sensation

¼ c. almonds
¼ c. oatmeal
3 Tbsp. cocoa butter, melted
2 Tbsp. honey

In a blender, process almonds until finely ground. Set aside. In the same blender, pulse oatmeal into same fine consistency. In a bowl, combine almonds, oatmeal, cocoa butter, and honey. Rub mixture onto feet, put on cotton socks, and leave on overnight. The next morning, remove socks and rinse feet in cool water.

Cinnamon-Sugar Scrub

1 c. sugar
¼ c. milk or heavy whipping cream
2 Tbsp. olive oil
Juice 1 lemon
Dash ground cinnamon
4 drops lemon essential oil

Mix ingredients using a whisk. Massage on hands and feet. Leave on for 10 minutes. Rinse with warm water.

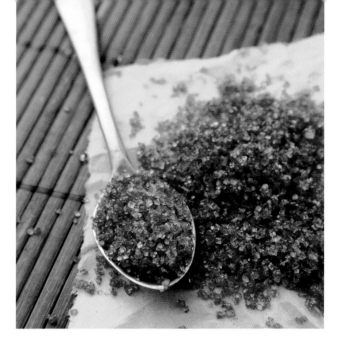

Walnut Exfoliant

½   c. walnuts
1   tsp. honey
1   Tbsp. olive oil
1   Tbsp. castor oil

Grind walnuts to a coarse powder. Add remaining ingredients and blend into a thick paste. Rub hands and feet with paste. Rinse with warm water.

Orange Lotion

2   Tbsp. orange juice
2   Tbsp. olive oil, warmed
1   Tbsp. cocoa butter, melted
2   drops orange essential oil

Blend ingredients until light and fluffy. Store in an airtight jar until ready for use. Apply to hands.

Vodka Soak

1   c. whole milk
1   egg
1   Tbsp. vodka
½   c. lemon juice
1   drop lemon essential oil

Blend ingredients well. Pour mixture into a large basin or bowl. Soak feet for 15 minutes. Rinse with warm water.

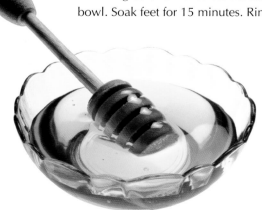

Toddy Wrap

½   c. brown sugar
½   c. spiced rum
Dash ground nutmeg
1   c. milk, heated
2–3 drops cinnamon essential oil
Moisturizing lotion (enough to coat hands)

In a bowl, mix brown sugar, rum, and nutmeg until the consistency of a scrub. Fill another bowl with warm milk and cinnamon oil. Soak hands in milk mixture for 3 minutes. Massage sugar scrub on hands. Rinse with warm water. Wet 2 hand towels with hot water and wring out. Pat hands dry and apply lotion. Wrap hands in towels and place each in a quart-size plastic bag for 5 minutes.

Honey-Lemon Hand Softener

2   Tbsp. heavy whipping cream
1   heaping Tbsp. cornmeal
1   Tbsp. honey
2   drops lemon essential oil

Combine ingredients well. Wash hands thoroughly; do not dry them. Massage concoction on hands, paying special attention to rough, dry areas. Leave on for 5 minutes. Rinse with warm water.

LEFT: Brown sugar is blended with spiced rum and nutmeg for the Toddy Wrap (see recipe on facing page).

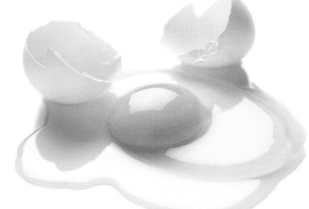

Foot Pamperer

- 7   c. water
- 2   c. milk
- ½   c. sugar
- 2   Tbsp. moisturizing lotion

In a saucepan, blend water and milk. Heat until mixture is as hot as you can stand. While it's heating, mix sugar and lotion until all the sugar is coated and mixture is slightly soupy. Put milk mixture in a large basin and soak feet for 10 minutes. Remove feet and rub lotion mixture over them. Place feet back in basin and soak for another 10 minutes. Rinse.

Avocado-Banana Pedicure

- 1   avocado, peeled and seeded
- 1   banana, peeled
- ½   c. sugar (the coarser the better)
- 3   Tbsp. sea salt
- 1   Tbsp. cornmeal
- 5   Tbsp. olive oil
- 2   Tbsp. plain yogurt or sour cream
- Milk (as needed)
- 10   drops essential oil of your choice

Mash avocado and banana. Stir in sugar, salt, and cornmeal. Add olive oil and yogurt or sour cream. Slowly stir in milk until mixture is slightly thick. Add essential oil. (If consistency is too thin, add more sugar.) Apply to feet and rub vigorously, especially on heels. Soak feet in hot water. When done, gently buff feet with a pumice stone.

FOR THE HAIR

Egg Shampoo

- 2   Tbsp. olive oil
- 1   egg
- 1   Tbsp. lemon juice
- 1   tsp. cider vinegar

Blend ingredients well. Shampoo and rinse well. Discard any leftovers.

Fruit Rinse

- 1   orange
- 1   apple
- 1   small slice melon, rind on
- 4   c. distilled water
- 4   c. cider vinegar

Peel and slice fruits, reserving peels. Puncture orange and melon peels with a fork to release their scents. Bring fruits and peels to a boil in water. Cover and simmer for 10 minutes. Remove from heat and let stand for 2 hours. Strain out solids and add liquid to cider vinegar. Pour in a bottle; wait 24 hours before using. Wash hair. Use 1 cup of concoction as a final rinse.

Lemon Hair Spray

- 1   lemon, rind on, chopped
- 2   c. water
- 2   Tbsp. rubbing alcohol

In a medium saucepan, place lemon in water. Boil until water is reduced by half. Cool, strain, and place in a spray bottle. Add rubbing alcohol as a preservative. (If mixture is too sticky, add more water.) Store in refrigerator up to 2 weeks. If your hair is dry, use orange instead of lemon.

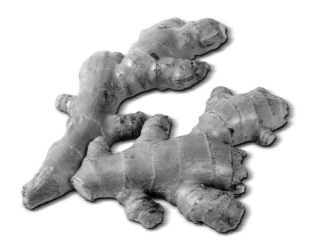

Ginger Dandruff Remedy

Fresh ginger root (as needed)
1 tsp. light sesame oil
1 tsp. lemon juice

Squeeze enough ginger root through a garlic press to obtain 1 tablespoon of juice. Mix with sesame oil and lemon juice. Apply to scalp and let dry before shampooing. Use 3 times a week.

Honey Conditioner

1 tsp. honey
2 Tbsp. olive oil
1 egg yolk

Mix ingredients. Massage on hair. Cover head with a shower cap for 30 minutes. Rinse and shampoo.

Strawberry-Banana Delight

3 strawberries, stemmed
1 banana, peeled
2 egg yolks
3 tsp. olive oil
3 tsp. honey

Blend ingredients and massage well into hair and scalp. Wrap hair in a towel. Leave on for 20 minutes. Rinse with warm water.

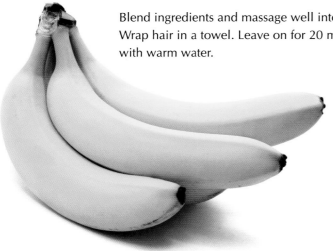

Apple Invigorator

2 Tbsp. apple cider
1 apple
2 c. water

Blend ingredients well, strain, and pour mixture into a bottle. Apply to hair after shampooing. Leave on for a few minutes, then rinse.

Tea Shampoo

¼ c. your favorite herbal tea, strongly brewed
1 c. liquid castile soap

In a saucepan, mix tea and soap. Stir over low heat until well blended. Cool. Store in a capped bottle until ready to use.

Mayonnaise-Margarine Conditioner

½ c. mayonnaise
1 Tbsp. soft margarine
1 egg yolk
2 tsp. wheat germ oil

Whip ingredients. Apply liberally to hair and scalp. Soak a terry-lined shower cap in hot water, wring out, and put on head. Leave cap on for 30 to 45 minutes. Remove and wash out residual conditioner.

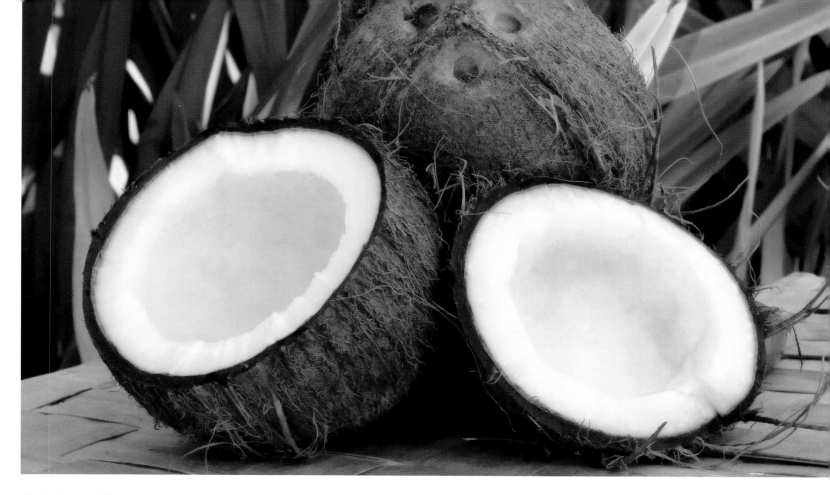

Fruit Smoothie

½   banana, peeled
¼   avocado, peeled and seeded
¼   cantaloupe, peeled and seeded
1   Tbsp. olive oil
2   Tbsp. yogurt

Blend ingredients until smooth. Apply to damp hair. Leave on for 20 minutes. Rinse.

Beer Rinse

2   Tbsp. beer (stale works fine)
2   Tbsp. distilled water
2   tsp. cider vinegar
5   drops rosemary essential oil
5   drops calendula essential oil
7   drops lemon essential oil

Mix ingredients. Shampoo hair. Use concoction as a final rinse.

Sesame-Coconut Conditioner

2   Tbsp. olive oil
2   Tbsp. light sesame oil
2   whole eggs
2   Tbsp. coconut milk
2   Tbsp. honey
1   tsp. coconut oil

Mix ingredients well. Massage into hair. Let stand for 15 minutes, then rinse with warm water.

ABOVE: The ubiquitous coconut yields both milk and oil for the Sesame-Coconut Conditioner (see recipe on this page).

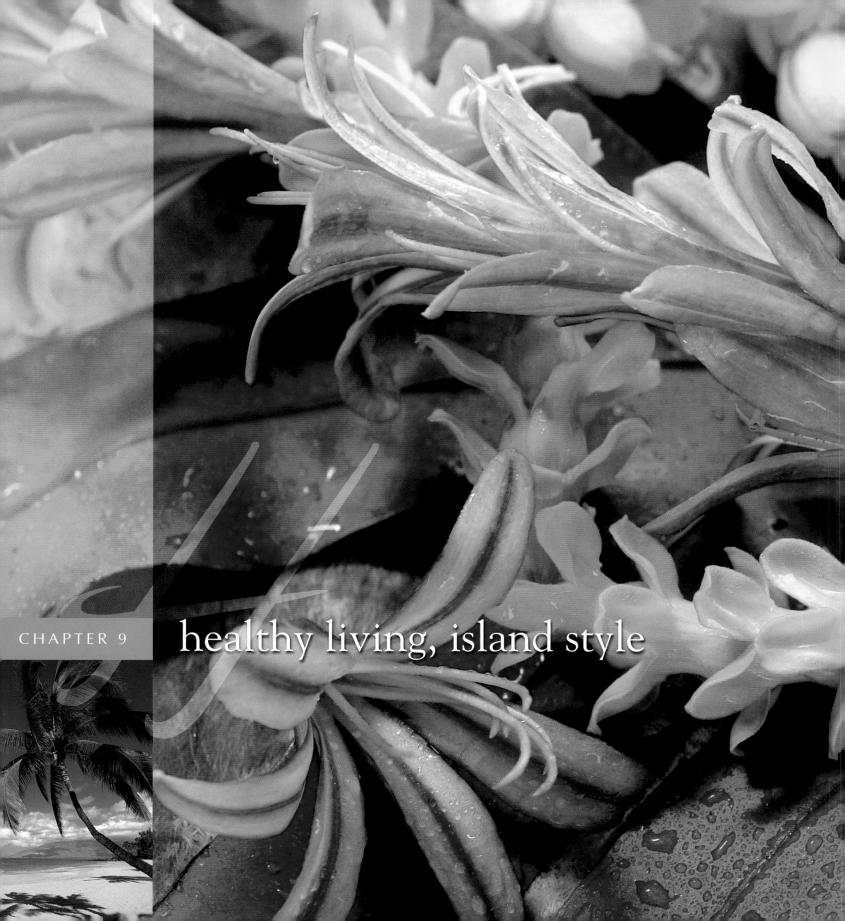

healthy living, island style

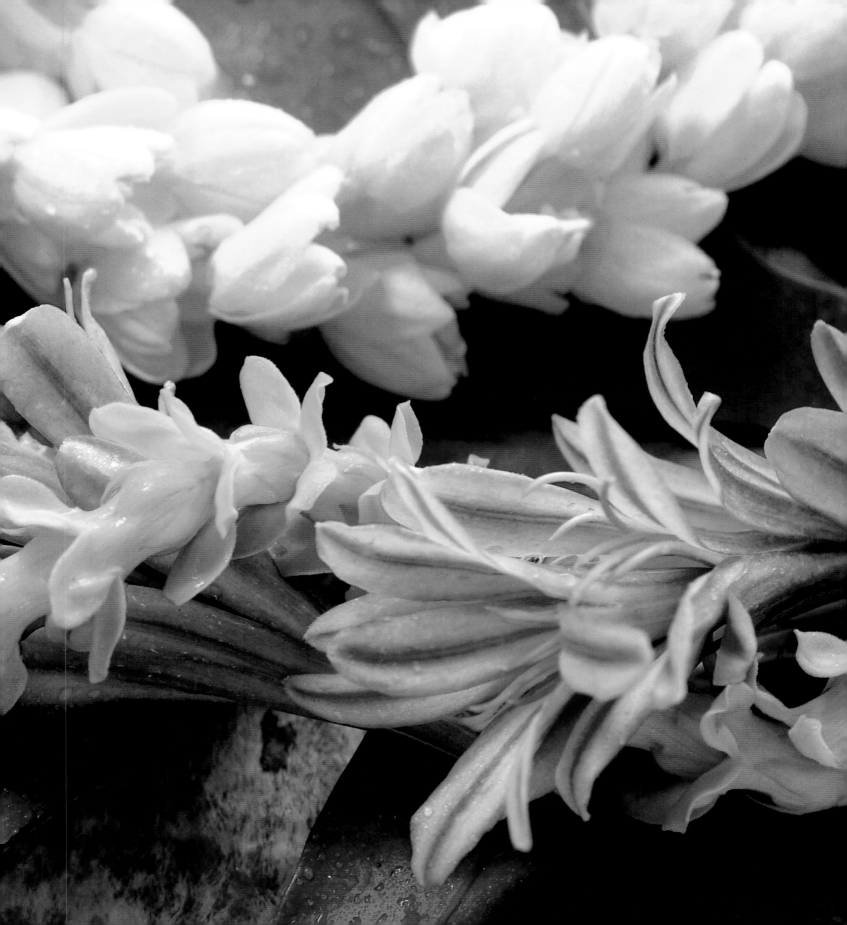

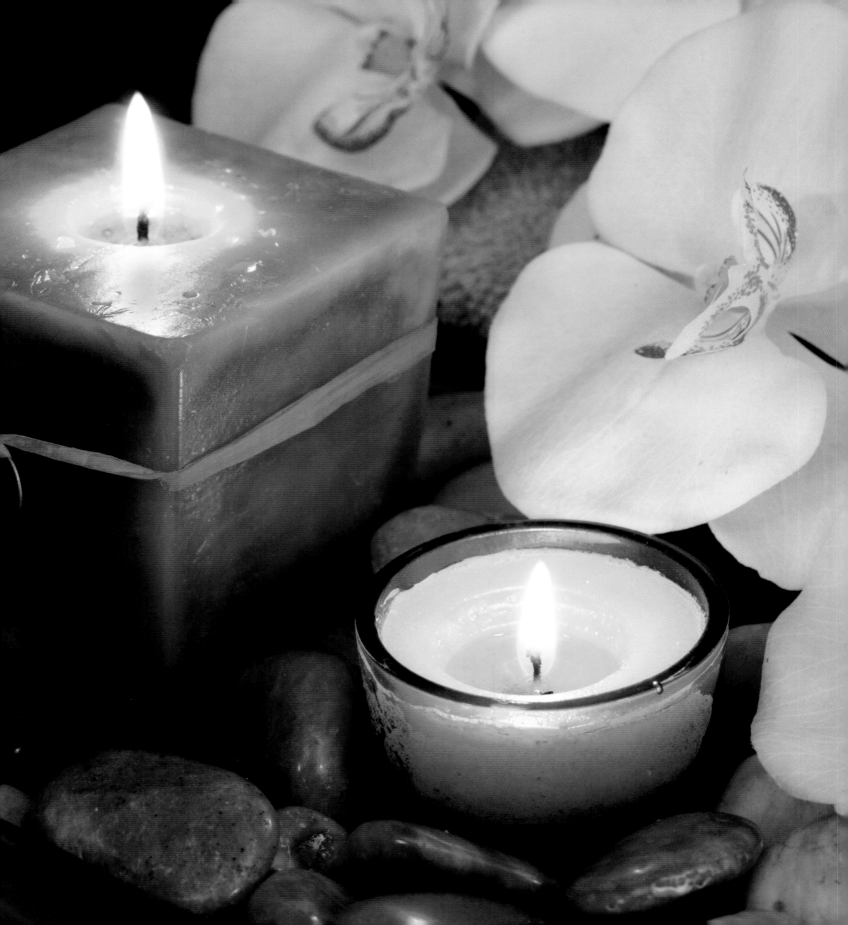

c h a p t e r   9

Attaining a healthy body, mind, and spirit may require making a lifetime commitment to major lifestyle changes. The following resources can be valuable guides on your journey to complete well-being. These resources are provided as a service; including them here does not indicate the author's or the publisher's endorsement of the people, products, events, retail outlets, or other listings, and does not guarantee they will provide the information or produce the results you seek. Also, this list is by no means complete; you no doubt will explore many other paths on your healing journey.

Holistic Centers and Wellness Retreats

O'ahu

Detox Retreat Center of Hawai'i
(808) 988-0800
www.detoxhawaii.com

Hawai'i Wellness Institute
(808) 848-5544
www.hawaiiwellnessinstitute.org

PRECEDING SPREAD: From spa therapists to manufacturers of organic food products, Hawai'i's health professionals recognize the healing gifts of nature.

LEFT: Think of the close to two hundred resources in this chapter as candles lighting your path to total well-being.

Inner Fire Hawai'i
(808) 255-9839
www.innerfirehawaii.com

Kapi'olani Woman
(808) 535-7000
www.kapiolaniwoman.org

Mālama Ola
Wai'anae Coast Comprehensive
    Health Center
(808) 696-1490
www.wcchc.com

Manakai O Mālama Integrative
Healthcare Group and
    Rehabilitation Center
(808) 535-5555
www.manakaiomalama.com

Unity Church Healing Arts Center
(808) 735-4436
www.unityhawaii.org/wellness.html

Women's Health Center
The Queen's Medical Center
(808) 585-5330
www.queens.org

Maui

Blue Bamboo II
(808) 661-7200
www.bluebamboospa.com

Kahua Institute
(808) 572-6006 or (877) 524-8250
www.kahuainstitute.com

Lani'āina Wellness Center
(808) 875-4669
www.laniaina.com

Mālama Nā Pua Hawaiian
    Healing Center
(808) 244-9008

Mālamalama Farm & Center
(808) 572-0499 or (888) 248-7017
www.malamalama.org

Ohana International Institute for
   Nurturing Arts
(808) 876-0409
www.maui.net/~mahana

The Studio Maui
(808) 575-9390 or (866) 427-1427
www.thestudiomaui.com

Island of Hawai'i

Ahu Pōhaku Ho'omaluhia
(808) 889-6336
www.hawaii-island-retreat.com

'Aina Me Kalani
(808) 959-2258
www.healinginparadise.org

Akash Ayurveda of Hawai'i
(808) 331-2276
www.akashayurvedahawaii.com

Aloha Healing Retreats
(808) 965-1244 or (888) 967-8622
www.healthretreats.info

GaiaYoga Gardens
(808) 965-5664
www.gaiayoga.org

Hale Ola
(808) 965-8917
www.haleola.com
www.voyagetowellness.org

Hawai'i Naturopathic Retreat Center
(808) 982-8202
www.mindyourbody.info

Hawaiian Lomilomi Massage: A Native
   Hawaiian Art and Cultural Practice
(808) 324-4720
www.hawaiian.net/~kea/aunty.html

Inner Journeys Hawai'i
(808) 985-9240 or (808) 640-7134
www.innerjourneyshawaii.com

Kahalelehua: A Center for the
   Perpetuation of Hawaiian
   Healing Traditions
(808) 968-1881
www.kahuna888.com

Kalani Oceanside Retreat
(808) 965-7828 or (800) 800-6886
www.kalani.com

Kokolulu Farm
(808) 889-9893
www.kokolulu.com

La'a Loa Wellness Center
(808) 322-1876
www.laaloawellness.com

Lōkahi Garden Sanctuary
(808) 889-0001
www.lokahigardensanctuary.com

Māpuna Wai Ola Healing Center
(808) 324-7202

North Hawai'i Community Hospital
(808) 885-4444
www.northhawaiicommunityhospital.org

Pele Lani Retreats
(808) 965-1899
www.pelelani.com

Portal Inc., The
(808) 775-9822
www.theportalinc.com

Sanctuary of Mana Ke'a Gardens
(808) 328-8998
www.sanctuaryofmanakeagardens.org

Studio, The (Center for Holistic Arts)
(808) 775-9911
www.thestudioevents.com

Tara Center, The
(808) 333-2080
www.tarayoga.com

Tutu's House
(808) 885-6777
www.tutushouse.org

Wood Valley Temple
(808) 928-8539
www.nechung.org

Yoga Oasis Hawai'i
(808) 965-8460 or (800) 274-4446
www.yogaoasis.org

Kaua'i

A Center 4 Wellbeing
(808) 822-2686 or (866) 822-9355
www.acenter4wellbeing.com

Aunty Angeline's Lomi Kaua'i
(808) 822-3235
www.angelineslomikauai.com

Ayurveda Center of Hawai'i
(808) 826-6621
www.panchakarma.net

Kahuna Valley
(808) 822-4268
www.kahunavalley.org

Pure Kaua'i
(808) 828-0380 or (866) 457-7873
www.purekauai.com

Moloka'i

Hui Ho'olana
(808) 567-6430
www.huiho.org

Mainland

Hawaiian Healing Academy
(541) 488-5879
www.manalomi.com

Health and Wellness Events

January

Kaua'i Wellness Expo
Kaua'i War Memorial Convention
  Hall, Kaua'i
(808) 652-4328
www.inspirationjournal.com

February

Great Aloha Run Sports, Health &
  Fitness Expo
Neal S. Blaisdell Exhibition Center
  Exhibition Hall, O'ahu
(808) 528-7388
www.greataloharunexpo.com

March

Native Hawaiian Health Festival
Bishop Museum, O'ahu
(808) 224-8068
www.hawaiimaoli.org

Total Well-Being Expo
Hawai'i Convention Center, O'ahu
(808) 949-5939
www.totalwellbeingexpo.com

May

Hawai'i Shamanic Retreat
Kalani Oceanside Retreat,
  Island of Hawai'i
(512) 708-8888
www.trancedance.com

June

Body Mind Spirit Expo
Hawai'i Convention Center, O'ahu
(541) 482-3722
www.bmse.net

Hawai'i Healing Garden,
  Kaua'i Festival
Malama Kaua'i
(808) 638-0888
www.hawaiihealthguide.com

July

Kawehewehe Aloha: Healing
  Through Love
Outrigger Reef on the Beach, O'ahu
(808) 924-6007
www.outriggerreef.com

August

Hawai'i Healing Garden,
  O'ahu Festival
Waimea Valley
(808) 638-0888
www.hawaiihealthguide.com

September

Hawai'i Healing Garden, Maui Festival
Maui Community College
(808) 638-0888
www.hawaiihealthguide.com

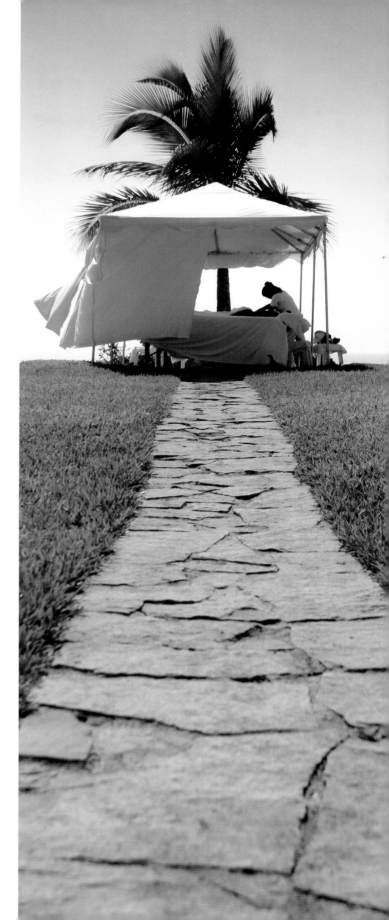

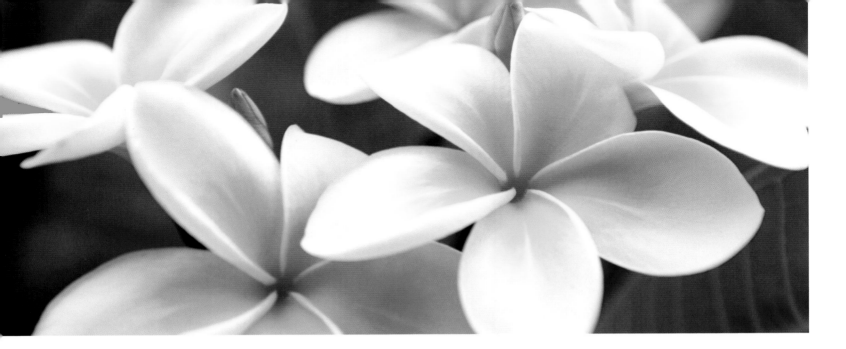

Total Well-Being Expo
Outrigger Keauhou Beach Resort,
   Island of Hawai'i
(808) 949-5939
www.totalwellbeingexpo.com

October

'Aha Lomilomi Conference
Amy B.H. Greenwell Ethnobotanical
   Garden, Island of Hawai'i
(808) 324-7202
www.lomilomi.org

Hawai'i Pacific Islands Kava Festival
University of Hawai'i at Mānoa, O'ahu
(808) 256-5605
www.kavafestival.org

International Health & Fitness
   Convention
Waikīkī Beach Marriott Resort & Spa,
   O'ahu
(808) 782-2161
www.fitpros.org

Mālama Ola
Grand Hyatt Kaua'i Resort & Spa,
   Kaua'i
(808) 742-1234
www.poipubeach.org

Voices of Hawai'i: Healing in the Spirit
   of Aloha
Pacific Beach Hotel, O'ahu
(808) 959-2258
www.healinginparadise.org

November

Hawai'i Healing Garden, island of
   Hawai'i Festival
Amy B.H. Greenwell Ethnobotanical
   Garden
(808) 638-0888
www.hawaiihealthguide.com

Unity Healing Arts Expo
Unity Church of Hawai'i, O'ahu
(808) 735-4436
www.unityhawaii.org/wellness.html

Health and Wellness Programs

Television Shows

Bodyworks
Oceanic Time Warner Cable
   Channel 16
(808) 690-5616

Cookin' with Cutty
Oceanic Time Warner Cable
   Channel 16
www.cuttytv.com

Get Fit Hawai'i
Oceanic Time Warner Cable
   Channel 16
(808) 781-7419
www.getfithawaii.tv

Hawai'i Health TV
'Ōlelo Cable Channel 52
(808) 225-1728
www.myspace.com/hawaiihealthtv

HMSA Now
Oceanic Time Warner Cable Digital
   Channel 344
(808) 948-5120
www.hmsa.com

Vegetarian
'Ōlelo Cable Channel 52
(808) 944-VEGI
www.vsh.org/tv/vegetarian-tv-
   Hawaii.htm

You can view past presentations online
at www.vsh.org/videos.htm (requires
high-speed Internet connection). You

also can watch the show online by going to www.olelo.org and clicking on Oahu 52 Livestream.

Wellness & Women on Wednesdays
Hostess: Sonia Chiyomi Fabrigas
Oceanic Time Warner Cable
 Channel 16
 Part of the Tiny TV show
Simulcast on *KWAI-1080 AM*
 (Honolulu, O'ahu)
 Part of the Radio Tiny show
(808) 524-8416

Your Total Health
KHON-DT2 Digital Channel 93
(808) 591-2222
http://tv.yourtotalhealth.ivillage.com

Radio Shows

Alive and Well
Hosts: Dennis and Mona Jones
KAOI-1110 AM (Wailuku, Maui)
(808) 244-9145
KQNG-570 AM (Līhu'e, Kaua'i)
(808) 245-9527
www.aliveandwellradioshow.com

Doctor Health
Host: David Snow
KHNR-690 AM (Honolulu, O'ahu)
(808) 533-0065
www.doctorhealthradio.com

Dr. Dean Edell
KAOI-1110 AM (Wailuku, Maui)
(808) 244-9145
KHVH-830 AM (Honolulu, O'ahu)
(808) 550-9200
KPUA-670 AM (Hilo, Island of
 Hawai'i)
(808) 935-5461

KQNG-570 AM (Līhu'e, Kaua'i)
(808) 245-9527
www.healthcentral.com/drdean/
 408/index.html

Dr. Joy Browne
KAOI-1110 AM (Wailuku, Maui)
(808) 244-9145
KQNG-570 AM (Līhu'e, Kaua'i)
(808) 245-9527
www.drjoy.com

Duke and the Doctor
Hosts: Duke Liberatore and
 Dr. Jan McBarron
KWAI-1080 AM (Honolulu, O'ahu)
(808) 523-3868
www.dukeandthedoctor.com

Healing and You
Host: Dr. Terry Shintani
KWAI-1080 AM (Honolulu, O'ahu)
(808) 523-3868
www.webhealthforyou.com

Health Smart
Hostess: Sherrie Rodi
KWAI-1080 AM (Honolulu, O'ahu)
(808) 523-3868
www.vimnvigor.com

Health Talk
Host: Hesh Goldstein
KWAI-1080 AM (Honolulu, O'ahu)
(808) 523-3868

Health Talk
Host: Dr. Ronald Hoffman
KAOI-1110 AM (Wailuku, Maui)
(808) 244-9145
KQNG-570 AM (Līhu'e, Kaua'i)
(808) 245-9527
www.drhoffman.com

HealthLine
Host: Dr. Bob Marshall
KWAI-1080 AM (Honolulu, O'ahu)
(808) 523-3868
www.healthline.cc

Healthy Body, Healthy Mind
Hostess: Dr. Diana Joy Ostroff
KWAI-1080 AM (Honolulu, O'ahu)
(808) 523-3868
www.naturalhealinghawaii.com

The Source Nutritional Show
Hosts: Damian and Karen Paul
KWAI-1080 AM (Honolulu, O'ahu)
(808) 523-3868
www.thesourcenatural.com

The Truth About Nutrition
Hosts: Rod Burreson and Mark
 Alexander
KWAI-1080 AM (Honolulu, O'ahu)
(808) 523-3868
www.roex.com

Wellness in the New Millenium
Host. Dr. Jason Uchida
KWAI-1080 AM (Honolulu, O'ahu)
(808) 523-3868
www.drjasonuchida.com

Wellness & Women on Wednesdays
Hostess: Sonia Chiyomi Fabrigas
KWAI-1080 AM (Honolulu, O'ahu)
Part of the Radio Tiny show
(808) 524-8416

Miscellaneous

HAWAIIAN HEALING FILMS

Zakwest Productions has produced three films on Hawaiian healing:

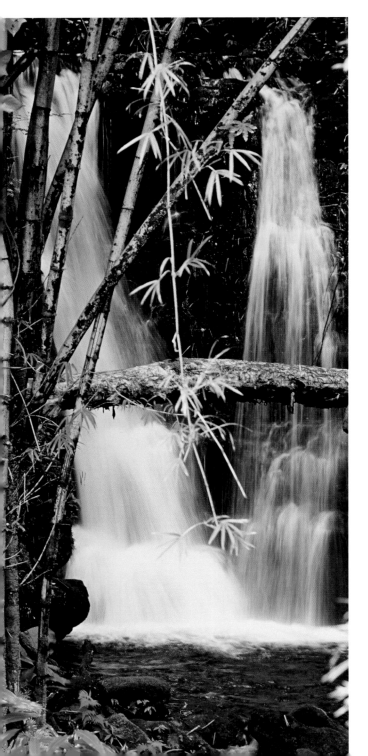

Hawaiian Healing, Hawaiian Meditations, and *Pule Wailele.* They are available on DVD at dozens of stores throughout the state, including Native Books/Na Mea Hawai'i at Ward Warehouse and Island Treasures Art Gallery in Kailua. They also can be purchased online at www.amazon.com. For more information, peruse www.zakwestproductions.com.

HEALTH CALENDARS

Listings of classes, lectures, film screenings, special events, and more (primarily on O'ahu) appear in the *Honolulu Advertiser's* Island Life section on Thursdays. The Shape Up column is a regular fitness-themed feature in those editions. Call (808) 525-8000 for details.

A similar calendar runs in the *Honolulu Star-Bulletin's* Today section on Saturdays. Health-related coverage in those issues also includes alternating columns—Health Options, written by local nutritionists, and the nationally syndicated Medical Journal, which discusses new studies and developments in medicine. Call (808) 529-4700 for more information.

Health and Wellness Publications

Big Island Body, Mind, Spirit
(808) 885-2181
www.hiwta.org/static/bodymindspirit.pdf

Hawai'i Wellness Directory
(808) 394-8438
www.hawaiiwellnessmagazine.com

Inspiration, Hawai'i's Wellness Journal
(808) 652-4328
www.inspirationjournal.com

Island Scene
(808) 948-5444
www.islandscene.com

Note: The printed version of Island Scene magazine is distributed only to members of HMSA (Hawai'i Medical Service Association). Non-members, however, can subscribe to Island Scene Online.

Maui Body, Mind, Spirit
(808) 214-7678
www.mauibodymindspirit.com

Maui Vision Magazine
(808) 669-9091
www.mauivision.net

Partners in Health
(808) 432-5932
www.kaiserpermanente.org/formsandpubs

Your Health
(808) 951-6790
www.yourhealthmonthly.com

Web Sites

Canoe Plants of Ancient Hawai'i
www.canoeplants.com

Five Mountains Hawai'i
www.fivemountains.org

Hawai'i Green Pages
www.hawaiigreenpages.com

Hawai'i Health Guide
www.hawaiihealthguide.com

Hawai'i Island Wellness Travel Association
www.hiwta.org

Hawai'i Medical Service Association
www.hmsa.com

Hawai'i Wellness Tourism Association
www.hwta.net

Hawaiian Huna Village
www.huna.org

Hawaiian Lomilomi Association
www.lomilomi.org

Holistic Association of Hawai'i
www.holisticassociationofhawaii.com

Holistic Hawai'i
www.holistic-hawaii.com

Kaiser Permanente
www.kp.org

Kaua'i Health & Wellness Association
www.kauaihwa.org

Lomi Hawai'i
www.lomihawaii.com

Lomilomi Massage
www.lomilomi.com

Papa Ola Lōkahi
www.papaolalokahi.org

Wellness Travel Hawai'i
www.wellnesstravelhawaii.com

Products

After Sea Aesthetics
(808) 876-0009 or (888) 923-8377
www.aftersea.com

Ahhhloha Bath Salts
(808) 836-8896
www.ahhhloha.com

Ali'i Kula Lavender
(808) 878-3004
www.aliikulalavender.com

Aloha Beauty
(808) 537-6937 or (800) 732-5642
www.alohabeauty.com

Aloha Sun Botanicals
(808) 876-1973
www.alohasunbotanicals.com

Berry Sweet Bath & Body
(808) 732-5100
www.berry-sweet.com

Essence of 'Īao
(877) 577-9343
www.essenceofiao.com

Hana Nai'a
(808) 936-8376
www.hananaia.com

Hawai'i Noni
(808) 247-6796
www.hawaiilure.com/catalog/
    noniproducts.html

Hawaiian Girl Botanicals
(206) 724-4057
www.hawaiiangirl.net

Hawaiian Islands Soapworks
(808) 281-6977
www.hawaiianislandssoapworks.com

Hawaiian Rainforest
(808) 683-1931
www.hawaiianrainforest.com

Hawaiian Rainforest Naturals
(808) 982-5989
www.hawaiianrainforestnaturals.com

Hawaiian Spa, The
(808) 233-8124
www.thehawaiianspa.com

Indigenous Soap Company
(808) 282-9084 or (808) 392-2409
www.indigenoussoap.com

Island Essence
(808) 878-3800 or (888) 878-3800
www.islandessence.com

Island Soap & Candle Works
(808) 828-1955 or (800) 300-6067
www.islandsoap.com

Ka'a'awa Soap Company
(808) 352-2145
www.kaaawasoap.com

Kona Natural Soap Company
(808) 322-9111
www.konanaturalsoap.com

Kopa Haiku
(808) 575-5435 or (866) 575-5435
www.kopahaiku.com

Kula Herbs Excellent Soap
(808) 242-0777
www.kulaherbs.com

Lanikai Bath and Body
(808) 262-3260
www.lanikaibathandbody.com

Mālie Kaua'i
(808) 335-5285 or (866) 767-5727
www.maliekauai.com

Maui Excellent
(808) 573-4005
www.mauiexcellent.com

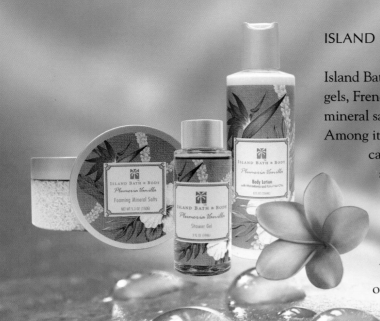

ISLAND BATH & BODY

Island Bath & Body offers a complete line of beauty products, including shower gels, French-milled soaps, exfoliating bars, body scrubs, bath sea salts, foaming mineral salts, body mists, body lotions, massage oils, perfumes, and colognes. Among its other products are scented and floating candles, hand-painted candleholders, sachet pillows, incense, silk cosmetic bags, and gift and travel sets.

You can find Island Bath & Body products at numerous spa and gift shops throughout the state, including Welcome to the Islands at Waikīkī Beach Walk (226 Lewers Street; phone (808) 923-4400). You also can purchase these items and more by calling (800) 468-2800 or visiting www.islandbathandbody.com.

Maui Lavender & Botanicals
(808) 250-2284
www.mauilavender.com

Maui Tropical Soaps
(808) 871-7667 or (888) 544-7627
www.mauitropicalsoaps.com

Mermaid Beauty Skin Care
(808) 283-9230
www.mermaidbeautyskincare.com

Monoi Tiare Tahiti
(808) 625-7728
www.monoi.com

North Shore Soap Factory
(808) 637-8400
www.hawaiianbathbody.com

Oils of Aloha
(808) 637-5620 or (800) 367-6010
www.oilsofaloha.com

Ola Hawai'i
(808) 959-2358
www.hawaiianbodyproducts.com

Plumeria Rain
(808) 391-4443
www.plumeriarain.com

Pure Hapa
(925) 818-0116 or (866) 900-6995
www.purehapa.com

Rainbow Ridge Farm
(808) 573-1675
www.rainbowridgesoap.com

Soap Box, The
(808) 284-6170
www.soapboxhawaii.com

Tropical Creations of Maui
(808) 572-0858

Waimea Body Essentials
(808) 938-3362
www.waimeabodyessentials.com

Warren Botanicals
(808) 334-1112 or (888) 848-0642
www.warrenbotanicals.com

Spa Accessories

Island Candle Company
(808) 637-8321 or (888) 646-6284
www.islandcandle.com

Kathryn's of Kona
(808) 326-4120

Kukui Nani Candles
(808) 634-0107
www.kukuinanicandles.com

Lomi Sticks by Ronald
(808) 286-3902

Maui Body & Soul
(808) 875-9004

Maui Magic Box
(808) 572-5551

Massage Supply Company
(808) 988-7033

Prosperity Corner
(808) 732-8870
www.prosperitycorner.com

Sedona
(808) 591-8010
www.sedona-hi.com

Serendipity Riches
(808) 949-4711
www.serendipityriches.com

Relaxation Music

Aloha Plenty
(808) 826-1469
www.alohaplentyhawaii.com

Dancing Cat Records
(831) 429-5085
www.dancingcat.com

Daniel Ho Creations
(310) 474-6507
www.danielho.com

Kahua Records
(808) 572-6006 or (877) 524-8250
www.kahuarecords.com

Mountain Apple Company
(808) 597-1888 or (866) 597-1888
www.mountainapplecompany.com

Palm Records
(808) 887-0107 or (888) 882-PALM
www.palmrecords.com

Wire & Wood Music
(808) 949-4411
www.wireandwoodmusic.com

Health Foods

O'ahu

Celestial Natural Foods
(808) 637-6729

Down To Earth
Honolulu: (808) 947-7678
Kailua: (808) 262-3838
Pearlridge: (808) 488-1375
www.downtoearth.org

Good Health Food Store
(808) 487-0082

Govinda's Vegetarian Buffet
(808) 595-4913

Hawaiian Kava Center
(808) 256-5605
www.hawaiiankava.com

Huckleberry Farms
(808) 524-7960

Kale's Natural Foods
(808) 396-6993
www.kalesnaturalfoods.com

Kava by Rex
(808) 284-1786

Kōkua Market
(808) 941-1922
www.kokua.coop

Marie's Health Foods-
  Organic Cafe
(808) 926-3900
www.marieshealth.net

Ruffage Natural Foods
(808) 922-2042

The Source Natural Foods
(808) 262-5604
www.thesourcenatural.com

'Umeke Market
(808) 739-2990
www.umekemarket.com

Vim & Vigor
'Aiea: (808) 484-4787
Honolulu: (808) 955-3600
www.vimnvigor.com

Well Bento
(808) 941-5261

Whole Foods
(808) 738-0820
www.wholefoodsmarket.com

Maui

Alive & Well
(808) 877-4950
www.aliveandwellinmaui.com

Down to Earth
Kahului: (808) 877-2661
Makawao: (808) 572-1488
www.downtoearth.org

Hawaiian Herbal Blessings
(808) 575-7829 or (888) 424-NONI
www.hawaiian-noniworks.com

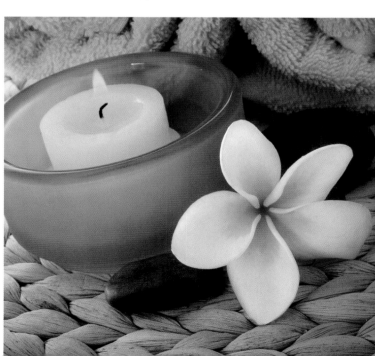

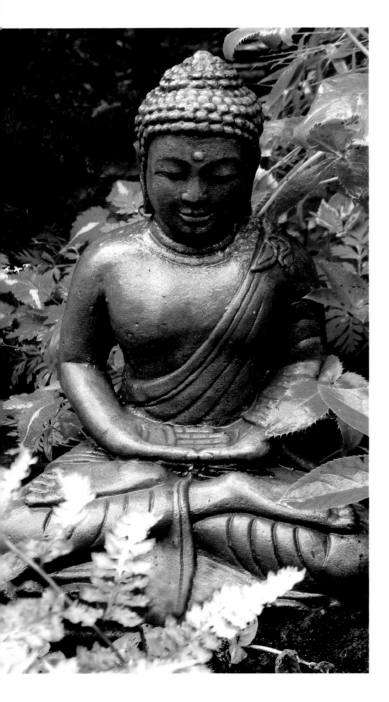

Hawaiian Moons Natural Foods
(808) 875-4356
www.hawaiianmoons.com

Mana Foods
(808) 579-8078
www.manafoodsmaui.com

Maui Medicinal Herbs
(808) 572-9331 or (800) 936-6532
www.mauimedicinal.com

Noni Maui
(808) 575-9100 or (800) 639-5454
www.nonimaui.com

Island of Hawai'i

Abundant Life Natural Foods & Cafe
(808) 935-7411
www.abundantlifenaturalfoods.com

Anuenue Natural Foods
(808) 929-7550

Healing Noni
(877) 662-4610
www.healingnoni.com

Healthways II
(808) 885-6775

Hi'iaka's Healing Herb Garden
(808) 966-6126
www.hiiakas.com

Island Naturals Market & Deli
Hilo: (808) 935-5533
Pāhoa: (808) 965-8322
www.islandnaturals.com

Kai Malino Wellness Center
(808) 882-1280
www.stevesullam.com/kohala.net/
   kaimalino/index.html

Kanaka Kava
(808) 883-6260
www.kanakakava.com

Kea'au Natural Foods
(808) 966-8877

Kona Kava Farm
(866) 649-2117
www.konakavafarm.com

Kona Natural Foods
Kailua-Kona: (808) 329-2296
Keauhou: (808) 322-1800

Hāmākua Natural Foods
(808) 775-7226

Kūle'a Farm Kava Company
(808) 959-5005
www.kickbackwithkava.com

Pu'u'ala Hawai'i
(808) 961-2888
www.puuala.com

Uka Kava
(808) 959-5282
www.mauikava.com

Kaua'i

Anahola Granola
(808) 822-5240
www.anaholagranola.com

Blossoming Lotus
(808) 822-7678
www.blossominglotus.com

Hawaiian Health Ohana
(808) 828-1123 or (888) 882-6664
www.nonifruitleather.net

ISLAND PLANTATIONS

Island Plantations carries six delicious flavors of island teas: Guava Strawberry, Macadamia Coconut, Mango Orange, Passion Fruit French Vanilla, Pineapple Papaya, and Tropical Tangerine. You can find these teas (as well as Island Plantations candy, cookies, biscotti, jams, jellies, syrups, and gift sets) at numerous retail outlets throughout the state, including Welcome to the Islands at Waikīkī Beach Walk (226 Lewers Street; phone (808) 923-4400). You also can purchase these items by calling (800) 468-2800 or visiting www.islandplantations.com.

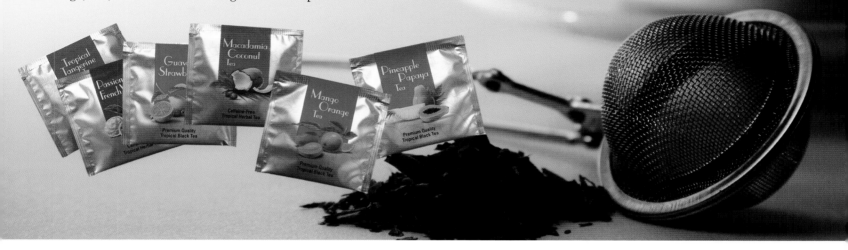

Healthy Hut
(808) 828-6626

Kaua'i Granola
(808) 338-0121
www.kauaigranola.com

Kava Kaua'i
(808) 821-1039 or (800) 626-0883
www.realkava.com

Kōloa Natural Foods
(808) 742-8910

Papaya's Natural Foods & Café
Hanalei: (808) 826-0089
Kapa'a: (808) 823-0190
www.papayasnaturalfoods.com

Vim 'N Vigor
(808) 245-9053

Moloka'i

Outpost Natural Foods
(808) 553-3377

Hawaiian Herbal Teas

Hawai'i Tea Factory
(808) 661-9401 or (800) 909-5662
www.hawaiiteafactory.com

Hawaiian Islands Tea
(808) 847-3600 or (800) 338-8353
www.hitea.com

Hawaiian Māmaki Tea Plantation
(808) 959-8185 or (877) 959-8185
www.organichawaii.com

Hawaiian Natural Tea
(808) 591-9400
www.hawaiiannaturaltea.com

Hawaiian Tea Company, The
(866) 652-2036
www.hawaiiantea.com

Maui Sun Herbal Teas
(800) 871-8817
www.mauisuntea.com

Pacific Place Tea Garden
(808) 944-2004
www.pacific-place.com

Traditional Hawaiian Teas
(808) 969-1604
www.hawaiianherbalteas.com

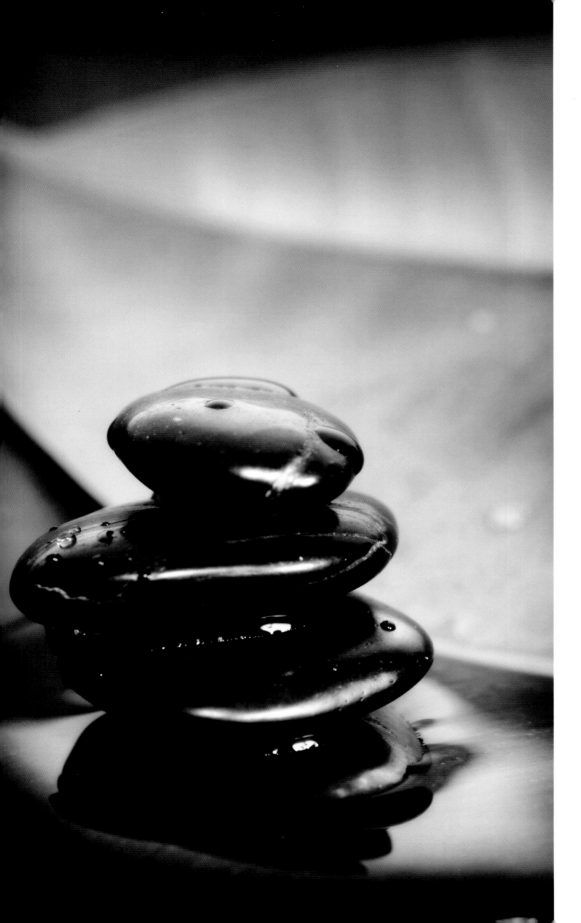

glossary of common spa terms

acupressure. An ancient Chinese healing technique of applying finger pressure on meridians (energy points on the body that correspond to different organs) to relieve pain and tension, promote relaxation, stimulate the flow of energy, and balance vital life forces.

acupuncture. An ancient Chinese healing technique of inserting fine needles into meridians throughout the body to relieve pain and tension, clear obstructions in the flow of energy, correct organ imbalances, and promote healing.

Alexander Technique. A method that corrects poor body alignment, releases tension, and improves well-being through awareness of the recipient's posture, breathing, balance, coordination, and movement in everyday activities to avoid or reduce physical strain linked to pain and disability.

aqua aerobics. A workout in a pool or the ocean that uses the support and resistance of the water to burn fat, strengthen and tone muscles, increase stamina, and improve cardiovascular health. Also called *aquacize.*

aqua bodywork. Therapeutic touching or manipulation of the body done in water. Also called *aquatic body therapy.*

aromatherapy. Treatments (including massages, facials, wraps, inhalation therapies, and baths) that use the fragrance of flowers, leaves, bark, seeds, resins, and roots to refresh, relax, rejuvenate, alleviate stress, and promote physical and psychological well-being.

Ayurveda. A traditional system of holistic medicine from India that uses aromatherapy, nutrition, herbs, essential oils, massage, and meditation to achieve total balance of the body, mind, senses, and soul.

balneotherapy. The therapeutic use of mineral, salt, or purified water (such as baths and thermal hot springs) to improve circulation, aid digestion, ease arthritis and gastric discomfort, strengthen the immune system, and relieve pain and stress. Also called *hydrotherapy.*

carrier oils. Base oils of a vegetable origin that are used to dilute essential oils, which are too concentrated in their pure state to be used directly on the skin. High in fatty acids, vitamins, and moisturizing nutrients, they provide the lubricant to transfer essential oils onto the skin. Common carrier oils include apricot kernel, avocado, grape seed, jojoba, macadamia nut, olive, sesame, and sweet almond. Also called *fixed oils.*

cathiodermie. A treatment using low-voltage electric stimulation in small doses to cleanse, regenerate, revitalize, remove impurities, stimulate circulation, and oxygenate the skin.

chakras. The body's seven energy centers located at the base of the spine, sexual organs, solar plexus, heart, throat, forehead (commonly called the "third eye"), and top of the head. According to Hindu belief, the chakras are all connected and must be balanced for a person to attain complete physical, mental, and spiritual health.

chemical peel. A chemical solution used to remove wrinkles, blemishes, and uneven pigmentation, and to smooth the texture of the skin.

chi kung. A Chinese exercise that incorporates movement, controlled breathing, and mental imagery to relax, strengthen, and energize the body. Also spelled *qi gong, chi gong,* and *chi gung.*

cold plunge. A deep pool of water maintained at a chilly temperature of sixty degrees or below. A quick dip here after a hot shower or sauna visit increases circulation and invigorates the body.

contouring. Calisthenics to tone muscles; increase flexibility; and firm up specific parts of the body such as the abdomen, buttocks, and thighs.

craniosacral therapy. The gentle massage of the head, neck, shoulders, and spine to improve function of the membranes, tissues, fluids, and bones associated with the brain and spinal cord. It also releases blockages in the flow of cerebral-spinal fluid in the spinal column to relieve headaches, back problems, and teeth grinding.

crystal healing. A treatment using the electromagnetic energy generated by quartz and other minerals.

Dead Sea mud treatment. Mineral-rich mud from the Dead Sea applied to the body to exfoliate and detoxify the skin, clean pores, relax muscles, and ease the pain of arthritis and rheumatism.

deep tissue massage. A firm, sometimes painful kneading of the muscles to eliminate knots, realign the body, improve posture, loosen muscles, release

emotional tension, and restore range of motion and freedom of movement.

dry brush massage. An exfoliating technique using a natural bristle brush to remove dead skin cells and impurities and stimulate circulation. Also called *brush* and *tone.*

dulse scrub. An exfoliating body treatment using a mixture of dulse seaweed powder and essential oil or water to remove dead skin cells and supply the skin with vitamins and minerals.

effleurage. Quick, long strokes usually used at the beginning and end of a massage.

electrotherapy. The therapeutic use of electricity.

Esalen massage. A modality embracing the philosophies that touching, caring, and awareness of the body are as important to complete healing as alleviating physical problems, and that healing comes as much from within as from the outside. Its basic foundation is Swedish massage, but it is influenced by Rolfing, Trager massage, Feldenkrais, meditation, yoga, polarity therapy, craniosacral therapy, psychotherapy, and intuitiveness to achieve relaxation, stimulate circulation, release emotions, renew vigor, and sharpen the senses.

essential oils. Aromatic liquid extracts obtained from flowers, fruits, herbs, grasses, leaves, seeds, roots, mosses, bark, shrubs, trees, resins, and spices for use in cosmetics, foods, and medicinal treatments such as aromatherapy.

exfoliation. The removal of dead cells on the upper layer of the skin to improve circulation and restore suppleness and softness. It can be done in a variety of ways, including using masks, paraffin, brushes, loofah sponges, sea salt, essential oils, or water.

facial. A treatment of several steps to relax muscles, soften lines and wrinkles, and revitalize and rehydrate the skin on the face and neck. It usually involves unplugging pores, extracting blackheads, cleansing, exfoliating, toning, massaging, steaming, and moisturizing.

fango therapy. A treatment using various types of thermal mineral- and nutrient-rich mud to cleanse, exfoliate, and nourish the skin; release tension; relax muscles and joints; improve circulation; relieve the pain and stiffness of arthritis and rheumatism; and eliminate toxins from the body. *Fango* is the Italian word for mud.

Feldenkrais. A movement therapy that combines biomechanics, psychology, martial arts, and physical pressure and manipulation to improve posture, flexibility, coordination, and self-image, and to alleviate stress and muscular tension and pain.

flotation tank. An enclosed tank measuring a little larger than a twin-size bed that contains about a foot of sterile body-temperature salt water. Treatment involves floating in this tank in quiet darkness to reduce stress; promote relaxation; and create the safe, nurturing feeling of returning to the womb.

glycolic peel. A preparation containing alpha hydroxy acid derived from citrus fruits to deeply exfoliate the face, which smooths the skin, softens wrinkles, evens pigmentation, and fades age spots and acne scars.

gommage. The application of various creams in long, massage-like strokes to cleanse and moisturize the body.

Hellerwork. Deep bodywork on the fascia (the sheet of connective tissue covering or binding together body structures) using fingers, knuckles, elbows, and arms to create suppleness and tissue mobilization so the muscles can move properly and bones can be held in the optimum position. It also improves posture; releases chronic tension and stress; realigns and balances the body; and increases energy, flexibility, and range of motion.

herbal wrap. A treatment that first wraps the body in warm sheets that have been steeped in an herbal solution, then covers it with blankets or towels to seal in the moist heat. It promotes relaxation, soothes soreness, softens the skin, opens pores, improves circulation, and eliminates toxins through perspiration. Cool compresses are applied to the forehead to prevent the body temperature from rising too high.

holistic medicine. The philosophy of health care that emphasizes the need to look at the whole person—including physical, mental, emotional, social, and spiritual aspects—along with diet, environment, and lifestyle values to create a program to attain optimum health.

homeopathy. A medical practice that treats a disease by administering minute doses of natural substances that produce symptoms similar to those of the disease, thus encouraging the body to heal itself.

hot stone massage. Smooth, heated stones of various sizes used with light pressure—in massage strokes or placed on different areas of the body such as on the back, in the palms, or between the toes—to relieve pain and stiffness and to restore energy.

hydromassage. An underwater massage in a deep tub using high-pressure jets and a hand-manipulated hose to stimulate circulation and alleviate fatigue, arthritis, muscle soreness, and joint stiffness.

hydropathy. A method of treating disease by copious and frequent use of water, both externally and internally.

hydrotherapy. The therapeutic use of water, including hydromassage, jet sprays, showers, baths, Roman pools, and whirlpools. Also called *balneotherapy*.

inhalation therapy. A treatment involving the inhalation of steam infused with medicine or herbal or mineral substances to alleviate respiratory, pulmonary, or sinus-related problems.

jin shin jyutsu. A modality based on the premise that pain and illnesses begin with energy blockages and disruptions, and involving lightly holding the fingertips on the body's energy centers in specific combinations. This restores harmonious flow and balance of energy, which alleviates stress and reawakens the body's natural ability to heal itself. The recipient remains fully clothed, and it is a painless procedure that doesn't involve massage, manipulation of muscles or bones, or the use of drugs or needles.

Kniepp therapy. A treatment combining hydrotherapy, herbal medicine, and a diet of natural foods.

lomilomi. Traditional Hawaiian massage characterized by long, continuous strokes and flowing, rhythmic motions using the forearms as well as the hands. It has been described as gentle waves moving over the body.

loofah. A sponge made from the fibrous skeleton of the fruit of the loofah, a tropical plant in the gourd family. It's used for a brisk full-body scrub that exfoliates the skin, stimulates circulation, and promotes relaxation.

lymph drainage. A gentle pumping massage technique around the lymph nodes to drain toxins and excess fluids, stimulate circulation, and boost the body's immune system and ability to absorb nutrients. It's effective for those who suffer from colds, arthritis, headaches, and sinus problems.

manicure. A hand treatment, including moisturizing, reflexology, and shaping and polishing nails.

mask. A preparation for the face such as a cleanser or mud mask that tightens as it dries to absorb dirt, exfoliate dead skin cells, and tone tissue.

massage. The manipulation of tissue (as by rubbing, kneading, stroking, or tapping) with the hand or an instrument for therapeutic purposes.

meditation. Contemplation, reflection, or mental exercise for the purpose of relaxing, achieving emotional well-being, and reaching a heightened level of spiritual awareness and connection with the inner self. Usually focuses on breathing and concentrating on a specific thought or object.

meridian. Any of the pathways along which the body's vital energy flows.

microdermabrasion. A facial exfoliation procedure that gently abrades the skin with ultrafine crystals of aluminum oxide. It reduces crow's-feet, wrinkles, sun damage, age spots, and acne scars while stimulating collagen growth and the production of skin cells.

mineral water. Water that has been naturally or artificially infused with mineral salts or gases, valued for its therapeutic properties.

moor mud. A peat preparation (usually referring to mud from an Austrian moor) containing biominerals; proteins; vitamins; plant hormones; and humic, amino, and fatty acids. It is used for cleansing; detoxifying; relieving sprains and inflammation; soothing aches and pains; and treating a range of skin conditions, from wrinkles and psoriasis to acne and eczema. The key difference between this and other substances used in spas such as clay, Dead Sea mud, or volcanic mud is that it is organic; the others are almost entirely inorganic, meaning instead of being derived from living things they are composed of minerals such as iron and calcium.

naturopathy. A system of treating disease that avoids drugs and surgery, instead emphasizing the use of natural healing procedures and agents such as water, herbs, and flowers.

oxygen facial. A treatment in which, after cleansing, steaming, and exfoliation, the face is sprayed with pure oxygen to diminish fine lines; prevent acne and blackheads; and stimulate collagen production, which is said to reduce the signs of aging.

parafango. A treatment combining mud and warm paraffin to detoxify, exfoliate, promote joint and muscle mobility, and alleviate aches and pains due to conditions such as arthritis and rheumatism.

paraffin wrap. Warm liquid paraffin infused with emollients applied to the body. As it cools, it solidifies, removing dirt from pores, removing dead skin cells, and drawing out toxins through perspiration.

pedicure. A foot treatment, including moisturizing; reflexology; and soaking, shaping, and polishing nails.

percussion. A massage technique of rapid alternating strikes to the body akin to light karate chops to relax tense muscles.

petrissage. A massage technique involving deep circular movement of the fingertips or thumbs on a particular muscle.

Pilates. A body-conditioning program that develops flexibility and strength without building bulk through breathing techniques and precise movements using specially designed exercise equipment. A routine of this gentle resistance and stretching reshapes and aligns the body, and improves posture, coordination, and concentration.

polarity therapy. A massage technique that combines gentle rocking, pressure on the meridians, and holding and stretching muscles to stimulate energy flow, promote relaxation, and achieve correct body alignment.

pressure point massage. Pressure on designated areas of the body connected to major nerves to release tension and strain. *Shiatsu* is a form of pressure point massage.

reflexology. A technique that involves applying pressure to specific points on the hands, feet, and ears that correspond to major organs. It promotes relaxation, releases blockages, improves circulation and lymph drainage, relieves tension and pain, and restores the flow of energy throughout the body.

Reiki. A Japanese technique that involves gently resting the palms on tense or injured spots of the body for a few minutes without movement or manipulation of any kind. Healing energy flows from the practitioner's body into the recipient. A calming, nurturing process, it aligns the chakras and activates and channels energy to organs and glands.

repaichage. A technique that involves applying a combination of herbs, seaweed, and clay and/or mud masks to the face or full body to cleanse and moisturize the skin.

Rolfing. A technique that involves very deep, sometimes painful manipulation of injured areas and massage of rigid muscles, bones, and joints to improve movement, balance, and flexibility; realign the skeletal structure; stimulate energy flow; and relieve stress caused by emotional trauma.

Roman bath. In ancient Rome, where it was developed, a bath in alternating hot, warm, and cold pools to improve circulation. Today it refers to a hot whirlpool or Jacuzzi equipped with benches for seated bathing. Also called *Roman pools.*

salt glow. A treatment that involves vigorously scrubbing the body with a mixture of coarse salt and aromatic oils to cleanse, exfoliate, improve circulation, and smooth and moisturize the skin. Also spelled *salt glo.*

sauna. A wood-lined room heated to 160 to 210 degrees with less than 10 percent humidity. The dry heat opens pores, releases toxins through perspiration, relaxes muscles, and softens the skin. Followed by a cold shower, the treatment improves circulation and metabolism, strengthens the immune system, relieves stress, increases energy and stamina, sharpens the senses, and provides a total feeling of well-being.

Scotch hose massage. A standing full-body massage by a therapist using a high-powered spray of alternating warm and cold water on pressure points to stimulate circulation, alleviate muscular pain, relieve tension, invigorate, energize, and cleanse the body.

seaweed wrap. A treatment that involves covering the body with a mask of nutrient-rich seaweed and seawater, then wrapping it in a heated blanket. The minerals, vitamins, and proteins are absorbed, revitalizing and smoothing the skin and restoring its elasticity. This treatment also detoxifies the body and increases circulation.

shiatsu. A Japanese massage technique similar to Chinese acupressure that uses finger pressure on the meridians to improve energy flow, ease pain and tension, revitalize and balance the endocrine and immune systems, promote internal healing, increase circulation, and generate a sense of harmony and relaxation. From the Japanese words *shi* meaning finger and *atsu* meaning pressure.

sports massage. A deep, penetrating massage focused on the specific muscles and joints used in the recipient's athletic activities.

steam room. A tiled room heated to 110 to 130 degrees and filled with wet, hot steam to open pores, eliminate toxins through perspiration, soften the skin, and relieve tension. A cold shower usually follows to close the pores, stop the sweating process, and decrease body temperature.

Swedish massage. One of the most popular massage techniques, requiring the liberal use of oil to perform several different movements, including long and gliding strokes, kneading, tapping, deep circular motions, rolling of the fingers, muscle manipulation, gentle slapping, and vibration. It improves circulation and flexibility; eases muscle aches and tension; promotes relaxation; and flushes the tissues of lactic acid, uric acid, and other metabolic wastes.

Swiss shower. Powerful stationary jets of water aimed at various pressure points on the body, creating the effect of an invigorating massage. The water temperature alternates between hot and cold to relieve tension and stimulate circulation.

tai chi. An ancient Chinese martial art and exercise discipline that combines meditation; slow, deep breathing; and graceful, methodical stretching movements and balancing positions.

tapotement. A massage technique that involves light, steady tapping on muscles, causing them to slightly vibrate.

Thai massage. A body treatment that combines gentle rocking, yoga-like stretching, and acupressure to align the skeletal system, ease muscle tension, and increase energy, flexibility, and tranquility. It is performed on the floor with the recipient fully clothed.

thalassotherapy. The therapeutic use of seawater and mineral-rich marine products that have curative properties, including seaweed, algae, and sea salt. It includes baths, masks, and wraps to cleanse, detoxify, rejuvenate, energize, and nourish the body. From the Greek words *thalasso* meaning sea and *therapeia* meaning healing.

Trager massage. A treatment that involves gentle rocking, shaking, stretching, and rotation and compression to realign the body, release tension from the joints, improve flexibility, and promote relaxation.

trigger point massage. The use of deep, sustained finger or thumb pressure on "trigger points" in the muscles, ligaments, and connective tissues, which manifest themselves through tingling, tenderness, spasms, cramps, sharp pain, dull ache, or "hot and cold" or pins and needles sensations. This muscular or "soft tissue" discomfort can cause headache, nausea, earache, sciatica, blurred vision, or equilibrium problems. Trigger point massage helps muscles to relax, enabling blood to flow into the affected area, which transports oxygen and nutrients to the muscles and carries away waste products that can cause fatigue and pain. Also called *myofascial release.*

Turkish bath. A bath that involves going through a series of steam rooms of increasing temperature and then receiving a rubdown, massage, and cold shower.

Vichy shower. Multiple overhead jets that spray warm water as the recipient lies on a table covered with a waterproof cushioned mat. It usually is used to cleanse the body after a wrap, mask, or exfoliating treatment, but it has benefits of its own, including reducing stress, hydrating, and improving circulation.

Watsu. A treatment performed in a warm pool combining massage, *shiatsu*, stretches, joint mobilization, yoga, and flowing dance-like movements to achieve deep relaxation, relieve pain and stiffness, and improve flexibility and posture. The practitioner supplies support as the recipient is cradled, rocked, and pulled in waist-deep water.

waxing. The removal of hair from the face, arms, legs, or body by applying warm or cool wax dipped in cloth to the area, allowing it to dry, then quickly lifting it off.

wet room. A room for hydrotherapeutic treatments such as Vichy showers.

whirlpool bath. A therapeutic bath during which all or part of the body is exposed to forceful whirling currents of hot water created by high-pressure jets to loosen stiff joints, relieve muscle aches, and induce relaxation. The jets often are aimed at specific pressure points.

yoga. The Hindu discipline that uses controlled deep breathing, meditation, and postures that stretch and tone the body to improve circulation and muscle tone; reduce stress; promote relaxation; increase flexibility, strength, and concentration; and attain unity of body, mind, and spirit.

Zen. The Buddhist philosophy that says enlightenment is achieved by intuitive insight and meditation.

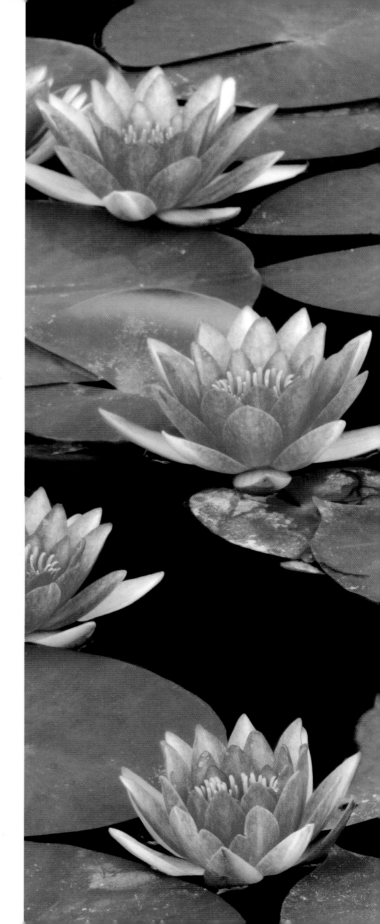

bibliography

Abbott, Isabella Aiona. *Lā'au Hawai'i: Traditional Hawaiian Uses of Plants*. Honolulu: Bishop Museum Press, 1992.

Avery, Alexandra. *Aromatherapy and You: A Guide to Natural Skin Care*. Birkenfeld, OR: Blue Heron Hill Press, 1992.

Bain, Joseph, and Eli Dror, eds. *Spas: The International Spa Guide*. Port Washington, NY: B.D.I.T., Inc., 1990.

Bardey, Catherine. *Secrets of the Spas*. New York: Black Dog & Leventhal Publishers, Inc., 1999.

Beck, Mark F. *Milady's Theory and Practice of Therapeutic Massage*. Albany, NY: Milady Publishing Company, 1994.

Boon, Heather, and Michael Smith. *The Complete Natural Medicine Guide to the 50 Most Common Medicinal Herbs*. Toronto, Canada: R. Rose, 2004.

Buchman, Dian Dincin. *Herbal Medicine: The Natural Way to Get Well and Stay Well*. New York: Wings Books, 1979.

Burt, Bernard and Pamela Price Lechtman. *100 Best Spas of the World*. Guilford, CT: The Globe Pequot Press, 2001.

Chai, R. Makana Risser. *Nā Mo'olelo Lomilomi*. Honolulu: Bishop Museum Press, 2005.

Chun, Malcolm Naea. *Native Hawaiian Medicine*. Honolulu: First People's Productions, 1994.

Clark, Linda. *The Ancient Art of Color Therapy*. Old Greenwich, CT: Devin-Adair Company, 1975.

Cohen, Sherry Suib. *The Magic of Touch*. New York: Harper & Row, 1987.

Cooksley, Valerie Gennari. *Healing Home Spa*. New York: Prentice Hall Press, 2003.

Crites, Laura, and Betsy Crites. *The Call to Hawai'i: A Wellness Vacation Guidebook*. Honolulu: Aloha Wellness Publishers, 2003.

Dodt, Colleen. *The Essential Oils Book*. Pownal, VT: Storey Communications, 1996.

Feltman, John, ed. *Hands on Healing: Massage Remedies for Hundreds of Health Problems*. Emmaus, PA: Rodale Press, 1989.

Fischer-Rizzi, Susanne. *Complete Aromatherapy Handbook*. New York: Sterling Publishing Company, 1990.

Gladstar, Rosemary. *Herbal Healing for Women*. New York: Simon & Schuster, 1993.

Griffith, H. Winter. *Vitamins, Herbs, Minerals and Supplements*. New York: MJF Books, 1998.

Gutmanis, June. *Hawaiian Herbal Medicine: Kāhuna Lā'au Lapa'au*. Honolulu: Island Heritage, 2004.

Heinerman, John. *Heinerman's Encyclopedia of Fruits, Vegetables and Herbs*. West Nyack, NY: Parker Publishing Company, 1988.

Joseph, Jeffrey. *Spa-Finders Guide to Spa Vacations at Home and Abroad*. New York: The Philip Lief Group, Inc., 1990.

Kahalewai, Nancy. *Hawaiian Lomilomi: Big Island Massage*. Mountain View, HI: I.M. Publishing, 2004.

Kaiahua, Kalua. *Hawaiian Healing Herbs*. Honolulu: Ka'imi Pono Press, 1997.

Kamakau, Samuel. *Ka Po'e Kahiko: The People of Old*. Honolulu: Bishop Museum Press, 1991.

Kloss, Jethro. *Back to Eden*. Loma Linda, CA: Back to Eden Publishing Co., 1995.

Krauss, Beatrice. *Plants in Hawaiian Medicine*. Honolulu: The Bess Press, 2001.

Lawless, Julia. *The Illustrated Encyclopedia of Essential Oils*. New York: Element Books, 1995.

Lazarus, Judith. *The Spa Sourcebook*. Lincolnwood, IL: Lowell House, 2000.

Leavy, Hannelore R., and Reinhard R. Bergel. *The Spa Encyclopedia: A Guide to Treatments and Their Benefits for Health and Healing*. Clifton Park, NY: Delmar Learning, 2003.

Lidell, Lucy. *The Book of Massage: The Complete Step-by-Step Guide to Eastern and Western Techniques*. New York: Simon & Schuster, 1984.

Maxwell-Hudson, Clare. *Clare Maxwell-Hudson's Aromatherapy Massage*. London: Dorling Kindersley, 1994.

McBride, L. R. *The Kāhuna: Versatile Mystics of Old Hawai'i*. Hilo: Petroglyph Press, 1992.

Meletis, Chris D. *Complete Guide to Safe Herbs*. New York: DK Publishing, 2002.

Mussett, Jennifer, ed. *Hands on Health*. London: The Reader's Digest Association, 1998.

Sarnoff, Pam Martin. *The Ultimate Spa Book*. New York: Warner Books, 1989.

Selby, Anna. *Aromatherapy*. New York: Macmillan, 1996.

Short, Linda. *The Complete Idiot's Guide to Self-Healing with Spas and Retreats*. Indianapolis, IN: Alpha Books, 2000.

Sims, Susanne. *Healing Vacations in Hawai'i*. Honolulu: Watermark Publishing, 2004.

Smith, Karen. *Massage: Simple Ways to Achieve Relaxation, Enhance Sensuality, and Enjoy the Healing Power of Touch*. London: Duncan Baird Publishers, 1998.

St. Claire, Debra. *The Herbal Medicine Cabinet*. Berkeley, CA: Celestial Arts Publishing, 1997.

Tierra, Michael. *Planetary Herbology*. Twin Lakes, WI: Lotus Press, 1988.

Tillotson, Alan Keith. *The One Earth Herbal Sourcebook*. New York: Kensington Publishing Corp, 2001.

Van Itallie, Theodore, and Leila Hadley. *The Best Spas*. New York: Harper & Row, 1988.

Wechsberg, Joseph. *The Lost World of the Great Spas*. New York: Harper & Row, 1979.

Wilkens, Emily. *More Secrets from the Super Spas*. New York: Dembner Books, 1983.

photo credits

COVER

Front: (foreground girl) ©iStockphoto.com/Miodrag Gajic;
    (background waterfall) Ron Dahlquist
Spine: ©iStockphoto.com/Amanda Rohde
Back (top to bottom): ©iStockphoto.com/Jacob Wackerhausen,
    Courtesy of Hale Hoʻōla Spa, Ron Dahlquist

FRONT MATTER

Page 1: Ron Dahlquist
Page 2: ©iStockphoto.com/Alan Crosthwaite
Page 5 (table of contents): ©iStockphoto.com/Liv Friis-Larsen
Page 6-7: ©iStockphoto.com/Ina Peters
Page 8: ©iStockphoto.com/Paulus Rusyanto

CHAPTER 1

Page 10-11: Jon Cornforth
Page 10 (inset): Ron Dahlquist
Page 12: Ann Cecil
Page 14: Peter French
Page 15: Peter French
Page 16: Ron Dahlquist
Page 19: ©iStockphoto.com/Ivan Bajic
Page 20-21: Vince Cavataio
Page 22 (clockwise from top left): ©iStockphoto.com/Matthew Scherf,
    ©iStockphoto.com/Ahmad Faizal Yahya, Peter French
Page 24: Ron Dahlquist
Page 25: Veronica Carmona

CHAPTER 2

Page 26-27: Ron Dahlquist
Page 26 (inset): ©iStockphoto.com/akaplummer
Page 28: Veronica Carmona
Page 30 (left to right): Ron Dahlquist, Ron Dahlquist, Donna Allison
Page 32: ©iStockphoto.com/akaplummer
Page 34: ©iStockphoto.com/Seth Loader
Page 35 (all): Ron Dahlquist
Page 37 (top to bottom): ©iStockphoto.com/Kelly Cline,
    ©iStockphoto.com/Brian Chase

Page 40: ©iStockphoto.com/Creativeye99
Page 41: ©iStockphoto.com/Feng Yu
Page 42: ©iStockphoto.com/Camilla Wisbauer
Page 43: ©iStockphoto.com/Sara Sanger

CHAPTER 3

Page 44-45: Peter French
Page 44 (inset): Jon Cornforth
Page 46: Peter French
Page 48: John C. Kalani Zak
Page 49: Peter French
Page 53: Courtesy of Kaʻanapali Beach Resort Association
Page 54: Peter French
Page 57: Peter French
Page 58: Michael Gilbert
Page 59: Paul L. Dyson
Page 61: IHP Archive
Page 63: Kiku Donnelly
Page 64: John C. Kalani Zak
Page 67: Val Loh

CHAPTER 4

Page 68-69: Ron Dahlquist
Page 68 (inset): ©iStockphoto.com/Fredrik Larsson
Page 70: ©iStockphoto.com/Yanik Chauvin
Page 72: ©iStockphoto.com/Elena Ray
Page 74-75: ©iStockphoto.com/Jacob Wackerhausen
Page 77: Courtesy of Hyatt Regency Maui Resort & Spa
Page 78: ©iStockphoto.com/Yanik Chauvin
Page 79: ©iStockphoto.com/Khanh Trang
Page 81: ©iStockphoto.com/Ye Liew

CHAPTER 5

Page 82-83: ©iStockphoto.com/Phil Date
Page 82 (inset): ©iStockphoto.com/winhorse
Page 84: ©iStockphoto.com/Nikolay Suslov
Page 86: ©iStockphoto.com/Fredrik Larsson
Page 87: ©iStockphoto.com/Fredrik Larsson
Page 88-89: ©iStockphoto.com/Marcela Barsse

Page 90: ©iStockphoto.com/Aimin Tang
Page 91: ©iStockphoto.com/Georgina Palmer
Page 92: Courtesy of AVEDA CORP.
Page 93 (top to bottom): ©iStockphoto.com/Natalia Bratslavsky,
    ©iStockphoto.com/Aimin Tang
Page 95 (top to bottom): ©iStockphoto.com/Julien Grondin,
    ©iStockphoto.com/Slawomir Jastrzebski, ©iStockphoto.com/ra-photos,
    ©iStockphoto.com/ooyoo, ©iStockphoto.com/James Margolis,
    ©iStockphoto.com/Christine Balderas
Page 96: Ron Dahlquist
Page 98-99: ©iStockphoto.com/Eric Hood
Page 100 (top to bottom): Courtesy of Hilton Waikoloa Village,
    Courtesy of Grand Hyatt Kauai Resort & Spa
Page 103: Ron Dahlquist
Page 104: ©iStockphoto.com/Kirsty Pargeter
Page 106-107: ©iStockphoto.com/Christian Michael
Page 108 (left to right): ©iStockphoto.com/Andrey Armyagov,
    ©iStockphoto.com/Galina Barskaya
Page 109: ©iStockphoto.com/Ferran Traite Soler

CHAPTER 6

Page 110-111: Courtesy of AVEDA CORP.
Page 110 (inset): Courtesy of Waikiki Plantation Spa, Outrigger
    Waikiki on the Beach
Page 112: Peter Vitale
Page 114: Peter Vitale
Page 115 (all): Courtesy of Mandara Spa/Hilton Hawaiian Village
    Beach Resort & Spa
Page 116: Tommy Taylor
Page 117 (all): Linda Deslauriers
Page 118 (left to right): ©iStockphoto.com/Jasmin Awad,
    Courtesy of Grand Wailea Resort Hotel & Spa
Page 119: Courtesy of AVEDA CORP.
Page 120: Jonas Mohr/J.M.E.
Page 121: Courtesy of Mauna Lani Resort
Page 122: Courtesy of Waikiki Plantation Spa, Outrigger Waikiki
    on the Beach
Page 123 (all): Courtesy of Grand Hyatt Kauai Resort & Spa
Page 124 (all): Seiji
Page 125: Courtesy of Four Seasons Resort Maui at Wailea

CHAPTER 7

Page 126-127: Courtesy of Grand Wailea Resort Hotel & Spa
Page 126 (inset): Linda Ching
Page 128: abhasa
Page 129: abhasa
Page 133 (clockwise from top): Linda Ching, Courtesy of Mandara
    Spa/Hilton Hawaiian Village Beach Resort & Spa, John C. Kalani Zak
Page 134 (clockwise from top left): Taku Miyazawa, Courtesy of Serenity
    Spa, Courtesy of Turtle Bay Resort
Page 137 (clockwise from top left): Courtesy of The Kahala Hotel & Resort,
    Courtesy of Waikiki Plantation Spa, Outrigger Waikiki on the Beach,
    Courtesy of Waikiki Plantation Spa, Outrigger Waikiki on the Beach

Page 138 (clockwise from top): Courtesy of The Westin Maui
    Resort & Spa, Courtesy of Luana Spa Retreat, Richard Wilson
Page 141 (clockwise from bottom): Courtesy of Grand Wailea Resort
    Hotel & Spa, Courtesy of Fairmont Kea Lani, Courtesy of
    Mandara Spa
Page 142 (clockwise from left): Courtesy of Four Seasons Resort Maui at
    Wailea, Ron Starr, Courtesy of Hyatt Regency Maui Resort & Spa
Page 145 (clockwise from left): Courtesy of Hale Ho'ōla Spa, Courtesy of
    Hale Ho'ōla Spa, Lia Watkins
Page 146 (clockwise from top left): Courtesy of Sheraton Keauhou Bay
    Resort & Spa, Courtesy of Four Seasons Resort Hualalai, Courtesy of
    Kona Village
Page 149 (clockwise from left): Courtesy of The Fairmont Orchid, Hawaii,
    Courtesy of Mauna Lani Resort, Taku Miyazawa, Courtesy of
    Mandara Spa
Page 150 (clockwise from bottom): Courtesy of Grand Hyatt Kauai
    Resort & Spa, Courtesy of Grand Hyatt Kauai Resort & Spa,
    Courtesy of ResortQuest Hawaii
Page 152: Courtesy of Sheraton Kauai Resort

CHAPTER 8

Page 154-155: ©iStockphoto.com/dashek
Page 154 (inset): Ron Dahlquist
Page 156: ©iStockphoto.com/Kelly Cline
Page 158: ©iStockphoto.com/Stefanie Timmermann
Page 159: ©iStockphoto.com/Ben Phillips
Page 160: IHP Archive
Page 161: ©iStockphoto.com/Djura Topalov
Page 162: ©iStockphoto.com/Jack Puccio
Page 164: ©iStockphoto.com/Sally Scott
Page 165 (top to bottom): ©iStockphoto.com/eliane,
    ©iStockphoto.com/Enrico Fianchini
Page 166: (top to bottom): ©iStockphoto.com/Marcelo Wain,
    ©iStockphoto.com/Angelo Gilardelli
Page 167: ©iStockphoto.com/pederk
Page 168 (top to bottom): IHP Archive,
    ©iStockphoto.com/Steven von Niederhausern
Page 169: ©iStockphoto.com/Gabriel Nardelli Araujo

CHAPTER 9

Page 170-171: Ann Cecil
Page 170 (inset): Ron Dahlquist
Page 172: ©iStockphoto.com/Pattie Calfy
Page 175: ©iStockphoto.com/Andrew Penner
Page 176: ©iStockphoto.com/Amanda Rohde
Page 178: Veronica Carmona
Page 180 (background): ©iStockphoto.com/Olaru Radian-Alexandru
Page 181: ©iStockphoto.com/emily2k
Page 182: ©iStockphoto.com/Shelagh Duffett
Page 183 (background): ©iStockphoto.com/Tomas Bercic
Page 184: ©iStockphoto.com/knape
Page 189: ©iStockphoto.com/Aimin Tang